CRITICAL ISSUES IN CHILD AND ADOLESCENT MENTAL HEALTH

D1344580

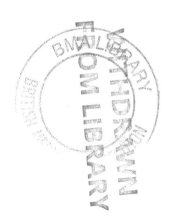

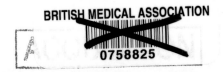

CRITICAL ISSUES IN CHILD AND ADOLESCENT MENTAL HEALTH

EDITED BY

SARAH CAMPBELL, DINAH MORLEY
AND ROGER CATCHPOLE

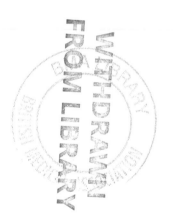

 palgrave

First published 2016 by
PALGRAVE

Palgrave in the UK is an imprint of Macmillan Publishers Limited,
registered in England, company number 785998, of 4 Crinan Street,
London, N1 9XW.

Palgrave Macmillan in the US is a division of St Martin's Press LLC,
175 Fifth Avenue, New York, NY 10010.

Palgrave is a global imprint of the above companies and is represented
throughout the world.

Palgrave® and Macmillan® are registered trademarks in the United States,
the United Kingdom, Europe and other countries.

ISBN 978–1–137–54746–0 paperback

This book is printed on paper suitable for recycling and made from fully
managed and sustained forest sources. Logging, pulping and manufacturing
processes are expected to conform to the environmental regulations of the
country of origin.

A catalogue record for this book is available from the British Library.

A catalog record for this book is available from the Library of Congress.

CONTENTS

INTRODUCTION

Critical reflection is a core academic ability. In children and young people's mental health, it is also a key component of effective practice. Mental health, or its absence, is the result of a complex tapestry of biological, social and psychological factors impacting on individuals over time. Practitioners in children's mental health come from a range of backgrounds and with different professional trainings in health, education, social care, psychology and other disciplines. That mix offers potential for deep insights and enlightened services, but also the risk of sterile squabbling over which is right or wrong. The capacity to remain curious and to consider the value to our understanding of ideas, evidence and theory emanating from perspectives very different from our own is a key skill for those studying and working in the field. Sometimes the most important thing is not the answer, but the ability to ask the right question.

In putting together this collection of writings, we have sought to raise some of those questions and to challenge some of the prevailing ideas that provide the raison d'être for the current child and adolescent mental health service (CAMHS) structure. We hope readers will respond thoughtfully to these challenges and consider how they might fit with their perspective, or generate new thinking leading to change in the way services are provided.

Each chapter is the work of an experienced professional from the CAMHS field or from associated disciplines. The authors do not always agree with one another. If we were able to gather them all together in one room, it is safe to say there would be a lively discussion between them – but what a seminar that would be. And this is the point of this collection of writings. Readers are invited to look critically at the material offered and, thinking about their own experience – and perhaps with the benefit of their own intuition – consider the ideas and arguments that are put forward.

The book does not, and perhaps cannot in a single volume, address every aspect of CAMHS. Inevitably we have been selective and are very aware that there are many topics – co-production with young people; gender and sexuality issues; and parental voice to name but three – which would merit chapters in their own right and could perhaps form the kernel of a future volume. Much of the content is, as the title implies, critical. But several authors also offer a vision of what could be and invite readers to address the question 'why not?'. A range of styles is represented and we believe that this offers a richness of approach. Some chapters are densely referenced while others are more openly polemical in style, but each presents a coherent set of arguments grounded in extensive experience of the topic.

We believe the book offers a thought-provoking read that encourages a reflexive appraisal of existing practice. As such, we hope it will cause readers to reflect on their own stance and ways of working and encourage them to question and improve the way in which CAMH services are delivered.

The first chapter by *Peter Wilson* critiques the robustness of what we have come to rely on as 'the evidence base'. He asks the reader to examine the 'givens' behind the evidence and cautions against its wholesale acceptance. At a time when so much policy, strategy and practice in CAMH is driven by the requirement to focus on 'what works', Wilson's challenge is fundamental. The second chapter by *Sami Timimi* challenges another core tenet of service provision – the organisation of child mental health services around given diagnoses. He argues that a much more nuanced approach to treatment is necessary to deliver person-centred care.

Matt Woolgar and Carmen Pinto critically examine the place of neuroscience in explaining mental health development in the child and young person. They caution against making claims for 'brain science' that may not be borne out by further enquiry and remind us of the dangers of over-simplification in the face of the real-world complexity of any individual young person's developmental pathway. In the next chapter, *Robin Balbernie* sets out the case for a much greater and better resourced focus on the mother and baby dyad. He explores the attachment framework, epigenetics and their effect on the mind of the developing child and suggests what an effective perinatal mental health service could look like.

Sebastian Kraemer's chapter illustrates the importance of meeting the psychological as well as the physical needs of children with illness and the value of access to CAMHS for paediatricians. Through a case study approach, he shows how collaboration between paediatrician and psychiatrist can positively affect the outcomes for the child. *Louise Richards* documents her personal, professional journey towards a sophisticated and nuanced understanding of the controversial diagnoses of ADHD and conduct disorder, tackling directly the evidence and argument around the increasing use of stimulant medication in children and young people.

Steven Walker's chapter on cultural context considers the way in which culture affects professionals' assessments in child and adolescent mental health services. Walker draws attention to the continuing evidence that practitioners ascribe explanations for behaviour based on their own preconceptions of both culture and gender issues. In an extension of this theme, *Dinah Morley* focuses on the specific issue of mixed race. The default position for children of mixed race is almost always 'black' and does not reflect the way in which these young people see themselves or want to be seen. Hence problems may arise in relation to identity and conflicting loyalties as these young people struggle to determine who they are.

Neil Humphrey draws on extensive research to explore the role of schools in promoting the mental health of children and the potential within the school system for effective early identification and intervention. He identifies factors key to effective implementation of universal and targeted interventions and elements likely to affect their success or failure in school.

Nick Barnes argues for a move away from clinic-based practice towards an approach that reaches out into the community and that is sufficiently scaffolded to remain safe and robust. Building on learning from his own work with schools and wider community based initiatives he describes a radically different model for CAMHS.

The book concludes with a chapter by *Sarah Campbell and Jenny Cobb* on what is perhaps *the* most important facet of the work – the therapeutic relationship. They argue that the resource pressures that are on CAMHS mean that practitioners increasingly have to curtail best practice, leaving them unable to develop the relationships with children that are at the core of practice in this field. Time for supervision, reflection and learning may be squeezed out in order to comply with contracts and manage within budgets with the result that the child is no longer at the centre.

We hope that readers will be enjoyably challenged by the contents of this book and will be spurred on to reconsider some of the pressing CAMH issues of our time. Whether readers are in managerial positions, working as commissioners or just starting out in practice, this book offers food for thought and a caution against taking some of the current 'givens' at face value without that all important critical reflection.

ABOUT THE AUTHORS

Robin Balbernie

Robin Balbernie is clinical director of PIP UK, a charity dedicated to help establish parent–infant projects across the country (www.pipuk.org.uk). Previously he was Consultant Child and Adolescent Psychotherapist in Gloucestershire CAMHS and Professional Lead for the Child Psychotherapy service. For over a decade, beginning with the Sure Start programme, he worked with the Children's Centres in the county as clinical lead of the team providing an infant mental health service, known locally and nationally as 'Secure Start'. He was also involved with the Intensive Baby Care Unit at Gloucester Royal Hospital and ran supervision groups for Health Visitors for 25 years. His interest in working with adopted children led him to the field of Infant Mental Health and early preventative intervention; and this became his speciality following a Winston Churchill Memorial Trust Travelling Fellowship to look at related projects in America. He is an advisor to the Association of Infant Mental Health, was a member of the YoungMinds' Policy and Strategy Advisory Group and a member of the APPG perinatal enquiry that led to the report 'Raising Greater Britons' (www.wavetrust.org/our-work/publications/reports/building-great-britons).

Nick Barnes

Nick Barnes has worked as a young people's psychiatrist within the London Borough of Haringey for over 15 years. Over this time he has worked in both generic CAMHS teams, as well as outreach services where there are significant concerns about the emotional wellbeing and mental health of the young person. He has also worked in paediatric liaison services, exploring the impact of long-term physical health needs on the child's emotional wellbeing. Having also been accredited as a cognitive analytic therapy practitioner, Nick often utilises this training in offering individual, parent or group-based interventions. However, much of Nick's practice within the community has been informed by 20 years of involvement in the voluntary youth sector within Waltham Forest – being responsible for running groups and camps for young people, both within the United Kingdom and across Europe. Recently Nick was also made Honorary Senior Lecturer at University College London through which he has been particularly involved in developing programmes around peer mentoring and initiatives contributing to the building of resilience within communities.

Sarah Campbell

Sarah Campbell is a Senior Lecturer at City University London where she is programme director for MSc programmes in Mental Health (CAMH and Adult). Sarah has completed and is involved with several research studies involving mental health and young offenders, child protection supervision and student nurse experiential groups. Having trained as a mental health nurse, she has worked within the NHS for more than 20 years and remains involved in mental health nurse training. Sarah is a psychoanalytic psychotherapist.

Jenny Cobb

Throughout her career, Jenny Cobb has worked closely with children and their families. Training as an RMN, SRN and CPN she was involved in developing services across a range of settings for children and young people and as a Nurse Practitioner worked directly with disadvantaged and displaced families. In her role as an academic and in partnership with YoungMinds, she helped develop a master's programme in inter-professional practice in child and adolescent mental health and as a Senior Lecturer contributed to the setting up of observational placements in nursery settings. Since 2001, she has worked as a psychoanalytic psychotherapist in both private practice and primary care settings and has gained considerable experience in supervising individuals and teams across the public and charitable sectors. She has a key interest in the emotional impact serial immigration has on the lives of children and their families and in the links between Bowlby's and Bion's early work on attachment and containment.

Neil Humphrey

Neil Humphrey is Research Director and Professor of Psychology of Education at the Manchester Institute of Education, University of Manchester. His research focuses on three areas: social and emotional learning, mental health and special educational needs (in particular, autism spectrum conditions). Neil's studies seek to move beyond considering 'what works' to instead ask, 'why various programs do or do not work, for whom and under what conditions they work, what is needed to scale up certain proven programs, and what policy supports are needed to scale them up without losing their effectiveness' (Slavin, 2012, p. xv). He is the author (or co-author) of over 120 publications, including books, academic journal articles and papers in professional journals.

Sebastian Kraemer

From 1980 to 2015, Sebastian Kraemer was a consultant emergency and liaison psychiatrist in the paediatric department of the Whittington Hospital, London, working in partnership with paediatric medical and nursing staff and with social workers. He is an honorary consultant at the Tavistock Clinic, where he was a consultant and trainer in child and adolescent psychiatry from 1980 until 2003. Besides paediatric mental health, he writes and lectures on family systemic therapy and its relationship with psychoanalysis, the role of fathers from anthropological and current perspectives, safeguarding and child protection, work discussion and professional development in medicine and mental health, the fragility of the developing male, early intervention, attachment and wealth inequality in social policy (www.sebastiankraemer.com).

Dinah Morley

Dinah Morley has worked in the health, social care and voluntary sectors. After working as a hospital social worker and then a primary school teacher, she joined the Community Psychiatry Research Unit in Hackney to run a community support team for people returning to the community from the North East London long-stay psychiatric hospitals. Following that, she became a principal officer and then assistant director of social services in an inner London local authority, finally moving to the national charity, YoungMinds, to establish the charity's consultancy and training service. She became the assistant director at YoungMinds and, prior to retirement, undertook the role of director for a year while a permanent replacement for the recently retired director was sought. Since retiring she has completed a PhD into the emotional wellbeing of mixed-race children and young people, an interest stemming from her personal experience and her teaching days. She is currently an honorary researcher at the Unit for Social and Community Psychiatry in East London and an honorary senior lecturer at City University. She is also a fellow of the Dartington Social Research Unit.

Carmen Pinto

Carmen Pinto is a Consultant Child and Adolescent Psychiatrist with the Conduct, Adoption and Fostering Team (CAFT), a National Service at the Maudsley Hospital that specialises in working with adopted and fostered children, and also with children presenting with complex conduct disorder.

Carmen has expertise in applying the biopsychosocial model of formulation to children that have been exposed to maltreatment and neglect and has developed this model in her service. She chairs a special interest group on the mental health of looked-after children for the Association of Child and Adolescent Mental Health (ACAMH) and links with national and international adoption organisations. Other areas of clinical interest are parenting, ADHD and attachment. She has an MSc in Clinical Psychiatry (University of Nottingham) and a Diploma in Cognitive Behavioural Therapy for Children and Adolescents (Institute of Psychiatry).

Louise Richards

Louise Marie-Elaine Richards has been working as a consultant child and adolescent psychiatrist in Hertfordshire since 2004. She also took on the additional roles of Named Doctor for Safeguarding Children, and training coordinator within her trust, and both areas have remained passionate commitments. Her interest in psycho-social factors associated with ADHD could be said to stem back to the 1980s when she worked for some years (initially as a volunteer) on a London HAPA adventure playground for young people with a range of special needs (including emotional and behavioural difficulties (EBD)). While studying medicine she ran trips and weekend camps for children living in women's refuges (from domestic violence) around the Manchester area. Her postgraduate training included a year working in paediatrics, before moving to London in 1995 to commence her General Adult Psychiatry training at the Royal Free Hospital. Having worked in both outpatient and inpatient posts across a range of disciplines, including general adult, eating disorders, psychogeriatrics, forensic psychiatry and child psychiatry, she went on to undergo specialised training in Child and Adolescent Psychiatry at the Tavistock Clinic, London (2000–3). Throughout her training, and since, she has remained fascinated by and committed to a range of therapeutic modalities, though particularly systemic and psycho-dynamic thinking and practice.

Sami Timimi

Sami Timimi is a Consultant Child and Adolescent Psychiatrist and Director of Medical Education in the National Health Service in Lincolnshire and a Visiting Professor of Child Psychiatry and Mental Health Improvement at the University of Lincoln, UK. He writes from a critical psychiatry perspective on topics relating to mental health and childhood and has published over a hundred articles and tens of chapters on many subjects including childhood, psychotherapy, behavioural disorders and cross-cultural psychiatry. He has authored four books, co-edited four books and co-authored two others.

Steven Walker

Steven Walker is an Alumnus of the London School of Economics and Political Science (MSc Social Policy and Social Work). Steven qualified as a social worker in 1985 and as a systemic psycho-therapist in 1992. After a career in child protection and child and adolescent mental health services Steven worked at Anglia Ruskin University where he was appointed programme leader for CAMHS. The course was judged *Most Innovative Multi-Disciplinary Training* by the Training Organisation for Personal Social Services in 2004. Steven has presented research at ten International Conferences and published ten textbooks and over 50 scholarly papers for international journals. His research interests include cyber bullying, military veterans' mental health and improving CAMH services for ethnic minority children. Steven is a UNICEF Children's Champion and member of the College of Social Work. Now semi-retired he still accepts work as an expert witness, is an external examiner at the Centre for Psychoanalytic Studies, University of Essex, and volunteers at a centre for unemployed people.

Peter Wilson

Peter Wilson is a Consultant Child and Adolescent Psychotherapist. He began work as a social worker in England and United States and then trained to be a child psychoanalyst with Anna Freud in 1967, qualifying in 1971. He has since held a variety of senior posts in the Camberwell Health Authority, Institute of Psychiatry, Peper Harow Therapeutic Community and the Brandon Centre.

From April 1992 until his retirement in February 2004, he was Cofounder and Director of YoungMinds. He has since served as clinical adviser to Place2Be. He currently has a small private practice and is actively involved in training at Place2Be and the British Psychotherapy Foundation.

Matthew Woolgar

Matthew Woolgar is consultant clinical psychologist in the National Adoption and Fostering Service and the National Conduct Problems Clinic, Maudsley Hospital, London. He was an academic in attachment theory and developmental psychopathology before training as a clinician. He has a particular interest in the assessment and treatment of complex presentations of adopted children or children from the care system, especially with regard to disentangling the effects of biological and neurodevelopmental factors from attachment, trauma and behavioural issues. His current research interests include the application of evidence-based parenting programmes to special populations, including adopted children, children in care and children with callous-unemotional traits. He also publishes on the identification and treatment of attachment disorders. Matthew Woolgar has had a long-standing research interest in the impact of parental psychopathology on infant and child attachment and the measurement of attachment security beyond infancy.

1

WHAT EVIDENCE WORKS FOR WHOM?

Peter Wilson

I am a psychodynamic psychotherapist. I have been one for over 40 years, working primarily with children and adolescents, having trained with Anna Freud at the Hampstead Child Therapy Course and Clinic (now the Anna Freud Centre) at a time when it was a centre of excellence in the training of child psychoanalysts.

I want to state this at the beginning of the chapter to give some indication of who I am and from where I come. Mine is, as is everybody's, a partial view – one amongst many that makes claim to its value in the broad field of psychotherapy. I am reasonably tolerant, respectful and, for the most part, curious about these other views. However, there is one particular view which simply bemuses and exasperates me, if for no other reason than that I see it as so intolerant of mine. I find myself sitting uncomfortably in the midst of what can only be described as a predominating scientific hegemony that seems intent to assert its supremacy in the world of psychotherapy on the basis of certain 'scientific' procedures, not least of which are random control trials (RCTs) and meta-analyses. Out of this stronghold, a firm belief has arisen that insists that psychodynamic psychotherapies are less effective than others which are supposedly better supported by 'the evidence'. Such a belief is increasingly being held by academics and policy makers. As Shedler (2010) observes, 'With each repetition, its apparent credibility grows. At some point, there seems little need to question or revisit it because "everyone" knows it to be so.'

I am of course wearily aware of what 'everyone' knows. Under the sway of this prevailing belief, I have felt from time to time inevitably buffeted and dismissed, both as someone who does not follow the ordained path and who, as a psychotherapist, persists in practising his own way of doing things. However, in recent years, in large part emboldened by those engaged in critical psychiatry and psychotherapy such as Sami Timimi (2002, 2007, 2013, 2015) and Del Loewenthall (2014, 2015), I have come to look more closely at the preferential claims made by scientists for certain psychotherapies over others that I favour. I have increasingly taken exception to the false certainties that lie behind these claims. In particular, I have discovered something obvious but so well camouflaged: that these claims carry the same kind of irrational bias and entrenched conviction of which I am accused.

As we all know, there are many pathways to the ever elusive 'truth' about the psychotherapies. There is a voluminous literature giving expression to all manner of psychotherapeutic ideas and approaches. All of them claim to be, in one way or another, useful and effective – and they all present their versions of evidence to substantiate their claims. The simple question then arises for me: what kind of evidence? There are of course many answers: some persuasive, others less so. But as far as I am concerned, what matters above all else is to know how far the evidence that is produced rings true for me – how far I can trust it to take into account the kind of psychotherapy I carry out. What I do is a highly personal emotional occupation – and I look to research that understands this and seeks to explore some of the intricacies and effects of what I and others do. Of course, I know that I am at risk of confirmation bias. But equally, within my own psychodynamic domain and through enquiries that are made within it, I find greater relevance to my own learning and development than bowing to the pronouncements of a scientific high ground that seems quite alien.

Choosing what's best for you

In November 2007, the child and adolescent mental health services (CAMHS) Evidence Based Practice Unit (EBPU) of University College London and Anna Freud Centre published a small booklet entitled 'Choosing What's Best for You: What scientists have found helps children and young people who are sad, worried or troubled' (CAMHS, 2007). Its intention was to inform young people about 'what scientists have found out so far, after comparing different ways of helping a large number of people'. It was widely distributed and is currently available and accessible on the website. I have no reason to believe its message has significantly changed since its publication. I have chosen to base this chapter on my criticism of this booklet since I believe it carries so forthrightly the fundamental values and assumptions of a dominant scientific community that is antithetical to the psychodynamic approach that I follow.

It is a lively publication, full of colour, bright cartoon images of smiling young people and, more, smiling doctors/scientists in white coats. It is well designed to capture the interest of young people and no doubt many others (including practitioners and commissioners – it is easy and quick to read!). So far, so good – here is a genuine attempt to reach out and disseminate the knowledge gained about 'what works'. However, once inside the covers, we begin to encounter in its structure and content a distinct flavour of partiality both in terms of its orientation and selected findings.

Its first two sections describe the different mental health difficulties that young people may have and the types of help that may be available. Unavoidably in such a small booklet, the descriptions are very brief, so much so that they border on caricature. The typology of mental health problems clearly derives from the well-known systems of psychiatric diagnostic classification. The main sections of the booklet are headed with several of these types in turn followed by guidance on which kind of help works best with each condition. Presumably, to heighten the popular appeal of the booklet, different kinds of help are star rated – three stars for those types of help that 'are very likely to help', two stars for those 'likely to help' and one star for those that 'might help'.

If we count up all the stars for all the conditions, we discover that medication is the most star rated, ahead of cognitive behaviour therapy (CBT) and way ahead of behaviour therapy and systemic family therapy. Other therapies hardly get a look in with very few stars. Psychodynamic psychotherapy scores just three stars; two for depression and one for eating disorders.

It may well be churlish to criticise this booklet. It was produced in the commendable spirit of a wish to share information gained from research with the wider public and young people especially. It drew on work contained in the second edition of a publication called *Drawing on the Evidence* (CAMHS 2006) again produced by the CAMHS EBPU, designed to provide 'advice for mental health professionals working with children and adolescents'. This in turn had been greatly influenced by a comprehensive review of the evidence published in the book *What Works for Whom? A Critical Review of Treatments for Children and Adolescents* (Fonagy et al. 2002).

There can be no doubt about the thoroughness of those who produced this work. Nor can it be said that they were unaware of the limitations of the evidence they were reviewing. They could see, for example, that different kinds of evidence show some treatments to be well backed by evidence and other therapies to be less so. Throughout the booklet, there are several 'reminders' to this effect. In so many ways, the writers of this booklet strove not to be prescriptive or directive.

And yet, despite their worthy endeavours, we have to ask ourselves whether or not they succeeded. Beyond their words and caveats, did they really convey the openness and fairness they sought to achieve? Did they manage to give a balanced view based on a wide range of evidence? Many thought that they did. But many, too, including me, simply greeted their publication with dismay and outrage. We could not comprehend how this booklet could be so narrow and one sided in its disregard for so much thinking at that time in building a comprehensive multi-disciplined national child and adolescent mental health service. Not surprisingly, the long-established psychoanalytic staff at the Anna Freud Centre, in which the CAMHS EBPU is based, were appalled to find that psychodynamic psychotherapy had been so minimally represented.

There were many other objections. Some were very concerned that a number of psychotherapies were not mentioned at all, for example the creative therapies (music, dance, art), solution-focused therapy, play therapy, not to mention the whole world of counselling. Some thought their forms of psychotherapy were poorly described or even demeaned as having no therapeutic value. Others objected to the rating system which they thought was crass, needless and unfair. Others thought some of the findings failed to fit in any way with their everyday experience.

Can it really be the case that this booklet was produced in the spirit of true impartiality, unaffected by emotional bias and irrational hostility towards the nature of psychodynamic therapy, at whatever level of consciousness?

The medical model: Diagnosis

Beyond all these various concerns, there is a more fundamental criticism of this booklet which relates to the values and beliefs that underlay its thinking – values and beliefs derived from medical practice. Throughout, there resides in its writing an unqualified commitment to the medical model of understanding mental health problems. Foremost in its structure is a basic focus on diagnosis and treatment. Clearly, from a medical point of view, this makes sense: ordering symptoms in such a way as to establish a basis for comparative analysis and to determine appropriate direction for treatment. Such an approach has served a useful purpose in the physical side of medicine. There are, however, many reservations when it is applied to psychotherapeutic practice. The question arises as to how relevant and appropriate it can be to apply such a model to the realities of everyday clinical practice carried out by a variety of helpers, the majority of whom are not medical practitioners.

For all the time and effort that has been put in over the years into the definition of psychiatric diagnoses in DSM (Diagnostic and Statistical Manual of Mental Disorders) of the American Psychiatric Association and ICD (International Classification of Diseases) of the World Health Organization, diagnostic labels remain by and large mystifying to many non-medical practitioners in the broad field of child and adolescent mental health. The ever-growing world of 'disorders' may make sense to psychiatrists and clinical psychologists, but for the most part it bewilders and confuses others so that they come to believe that there is something physically wrong with the children who worry them. The fact is that most of these diagnoses lack any clear 'discernible physical basis, any association with particular physical or biological tests' (Timimi, 2013). Psychiatrists base their diagnoses primarily on subjective judgement and evaluation of observable symptoms and behaviours rather than on the basis of any physical evidence. There is a clear issue of reliability here; it is not at all uncommon for different psychiatrists to make quite different diagnoses based on similar behaviour.

Many worry that the effect of such psychiatric diagnostic thinking is the medicalisation of ordinary human experiences. After all, 'anxiety' and 'depression', for example, are no more than fundamental human states of being; they are not in themselves pathological conditions. Psychiatrists of course will reassure us that these words are only used to describe conditions that are relatively severe and which significantly impair functioning. But a short hand tends to develop in the public mind so that distinctions are less clear. This situation is not helped by the fact that the psychiatric diagnoses as they stand simply do not capture the complex variety of difficulties that most children and adolescents present. The ever-abiding problem of 'comorbidity' confounds the tidiness of diagnostic categorisations. Within each diagnostic category there is such heterogeneity as to defy any kind of coherent understanding. Within the rubric of depression, for example, there is such a wide spectrum of disturbances ranging from mild forms of reactive depressed feelings to undeniably chronic clinical conditions. Similarly, 'anxiety' manifests itself in many ways, not least because of the many reasons that lie beneath it.

The medical model: Treatment and research

A major complicating effect of the establishment of psychiatric diagnoses relates to ideas about treatment. Because of their lack of clarity and precision, most diagnoses throw a confusing light on the paths of treatment that should be followed. To quote Timimi (2013) again, 'there is no evidence to show that using psychiatric diagnostic categories as a guide for treatment significantly impacts on outcomes'. Despite this, a great deal of effort has been spent on conducting trials and tests to assess the most appropriate treatments for different conditions.

Various forms of scrutiny of psychotherapeutic practice can be applied but the one that has been taken as the most objective and fair is the RCT – a clearly rational approach whereby individuals from identical backgrounds are allocated at random to one group which receives an intervention and another which does not. In this way, the idea is that a particular therapeutic ingredient can be isolated and identified. Once this is achieved, so the argument goes, a treatment can be directed. On the face of it, this makes sense and in relation to many of the medical physical therapies such as drug therapies, a great deal has been learnt for the good. However, can such a procedure be the right one to test a psychological therapy and most particularly a psychodynamic psychotherapy?

As supreme as RCTs are regarded and as influential as they may be in indicating the most effective psychotherapies, there exists a host of concerns about the way their researchers go about their business. These are thoroughly discussed in a paper published by the UK Council of Psychotherapy, 'NICE under scrutiny' (Guy et al. 2011). The National Institute for Health and Care Excellence (NICE) (2004, 2009a) was established in 1999 to provide guidance to health, public health and social care providers based on available evidence. According to NICE's guidelines manual in 2009, 'although there are a number of difficulties with the use of RCTs in the evaluation of interventions in mental health, the RCT remains the most important method for establishing treatment efficacy'.

The UK Council of Psychotherapy paper objects to NICE's methodology, which it believes 'has been inappropriately applied to psychotherapy'. It is seen as adhering to an overly medicalised perspective on emotional distress and 'treats psychotherapy as if it were a drug for research purposes when a more appropriate metaphor might be therapy as a dialogue'. It uses an inflexible hierarchy of evidence which its own Chairman has criticised. The chairman at the time of this paper was Sir Michael Rawlins, who said that 'to regard the randomized controlled trial as the gold standard is unsustainable' (Rawlins, 2008).

The fundamental objection to the rule of the RCT is that so many of its trials have been conducted in laboratory conditions, not in real-life clinical settings. This has been largely because of the need to control for research purposes the various variables involved in psychotherapeutic treatment. This is all very well in the tradition of experimental science and no doubt appropriate in investigating many of the physical treatments, such as drug therapy. In its application to psychological therapies, however, there is much to be desired.

For example, in most of these studies, in the researchers' desire to control the patient variable, they have been extraordinarily selective in deciding eligibility for the trials. In general, children selected for these trials are recruited through personal or professional contacts or through advertisements, rather than in response to clinic referrals. Similarly, the therapists employed in these trails are usually drawn from university departments with no specific or adequate training in the therapy under investigation. As a consequence of such rigid research discipline, many key factors that arise in everyday clinical practice are simply controlled out. The variable motivation of children is not taken into account, nor is that of families with varying kinds of worries about mental health, job security, economic status or the environmental conditions in which they live.

The training and particular beliefs of therapists as well as the pressures of working in contemporary community-based clinics are also not adequately considered.

Despite these serious reservations about the conduct of RCTs, the prevailing scientific view that permeates the research review literature and the booklet rests heavily on the evidence obtained from them. The fact that so many are laboratory based does not seem to disturb the confidence of those who hold this view. However, in a remarkably honest recent review (Weisz, 2014, 2015) it emerged that out of 461 youth RCTs that had been conducted during the last 50 years, only 2% were carried out in actual clinical service settings by practitioners treating children who were clinically referred and seeking treatment. This review was carried out by John Weisz, who himself has been actively involved with many of the RCTs that he reviewed. He could see, however, that laboratory-based trials did not take into account a range of highly relevant variable factors and as such their findings could not be successfully generalised into real-world clinical practice.

My practice as a psychodynamic psychotherapist

As a psychodynamic psychotherapist, I am left unimpressed, even incredulous that the RCT findings and recommendations that favour manualised, cognitive-behaviour-type treatments should hold such currency. CBT may have 'its place' (as they say) with some children such as those suffering from significant obsessionality and with others with moderate emotional difficulties. But to suggest, as the booklet does, that children suffering from anxiety, particularly at a severe level, are more likely to respond to CBT than the psychodynamic psychotherapy that I and others like me are doing is simply unconvincing. And am I really to believe, as indicated in the booklet, that meeting 'a few times' in systemic family therapy with a child suffering deliberate self-harm is really 'likely to help'?

What takes place in my consulting room reflects predomina who I am as a person and as a therapist. I come to my work with a set of beliefs and values that derive from my psychoanalytic training, my reading, my age, my gender, my emotional and social experience, my culture and above all what is engendered in me by my patients. Sometimes I am engaged. Sometimes I am confused. Sometimes I am scared. Sometimes I am angry. My therapeutic responses are not determined by some form of manualised diktat but rather by the way I process what I feel and think in my direct relationship with the patient, primarily through as much self-awareness as I can muster. Psychodynamic psychotherapy rests uniquely upon whatever kind of relationship might develop between therapist and patient. It is in effect a form of conversation arranged in such a way as to facilitate reflection and joint understanding. It does not comprise a set of techniques, pre-set and formulaic. I do not attempt to corral patients into some kind of conformist compliance. I do not tell patients what to do; rather I attempt to enable them to feel, think and find their own solutions.

This psychodynamic psychotherapy, moreover, is not determined by any kind of psychiatric diagnosis as such. Of course, I seek to make sense of the problems that are presented to me in terms of patients' current and past living circumstances. But I need to keep open about what might proceed in therapeutic work to ensure that I do not foreclose on what may later emerge of crucial importance. If, for example, I see a child who is miserable, failing to concentrate in class and finicky in her eating habits, I do not attempt to rush her into a diagnostic category that is so broad as to be meaningless. I am more concerned with finding a way of getting alongside her and gaining her trust as far as possible so that she can begin to share some of the feelings and thoughts that underlie her sense of disturbance. Similarly, in the event of my being asked to see a teenager who is underachieving at school and getting into trouble with the law, I do not hurry to categorise him as a conduct disorder but rather look for ways in which he and I can explore some of the preoccupations that may be getting in his way. And again, I do much the same with a teenage girl whose complaints of fatigue, inability to sleep and preoccupation with violent fantasies might in the first instance alert me to the possibility of an incipient psychotic process. I listen to her and to my own reactions and find a way in which she can feel safe enough to share with me her fears and desires.

Whatever commonalities may exist, there are significant differences between different psychotherapeutic approaches – but only some are favoured by the prevailing current scientific establishment. Throughout, the booklet trumpets the authority of the 'scientists' as if they carried some kind of divine oracle being so 'sure' of their assertions – for example, in the booklet, for a three-star type of help, the scientists 'are very sure about this way of helping'. Can anyone really be that sure of anything in the tangled and complicated life of psychotherapy?

So smug and lofty are these blithe statements that I find myself wondering, for the sake of comparison, what kind of a booklet might emerge if it were to be produced under the banner of something quite different, let's say that of 'the Artist'. The chances are that it would give us a quite alternative perspective and would draw its stimulus from a much broader range of evidences, lower down (but nevertheless, important) in the revered hierarchy of evidence, such as case-control studies, expert opinion and personal experience. It would in short include much that can be gained from practice-based evidence, from casework discussions, supervisions, published clinical papers and even from philosophy and literature. The chances are too that it would take into account other reviews such as Kennedy and Midgley's thematic review of child, adolescent and parent–infant therapy (Midgley and Kennedy, 2011).

Why does any of this matter?

On the basis of the prevailing scientific research findings, much of which is incomplete, inconclusive and methodologically faulty, major decisions are being made in public services to seriously and destructively diminish the quality of CAMHS and reduce patient choice. The recently arrived new programme, 'Improving Access to Psychological Therapies', IAPT (2010, YoungMinds 2015), is being imposed on the provision of CAMHS in many areas of the country. It is geared in the predominant direction of CBT and related manualised psychotherapies with the result that the posts of senior experienced child psychotherapists and others such as the creative psychotherapists are being 'deleted' and young inexperienced novices are being recruited in their place to conduct basic CBT work. This development, which is very dubiously called a 'transformation' in service development, is now forcefully underway. However, despite the assertions and protestations made on its behalf, it is facing questionable results. Timimi, for example, questions whether it is proving any better than what existed before (Timimi, 2015). Increasingly, reports are being made of inadequate therapeutic capacity to deal with the more severely disturbed young people – many of the new band of inexperienced recruits finding themselves frequently out of their depth, much to the cost of those they are supposed to be helping.

Conclusion

My intention in this chapter is not to complain about the demand for evidence but rather to protest against the overly influential dominance of just one type of evidence. My plea is that we need to open our eyes to the idea that different kinds of evidence suit different kinds of psychotherapies. I may well be accused, as a psychodynamic psychotherapist, of being arrogant, precious, self-congratulatory and resistant to any external enquiry. But equally those who fire these attacks are themselves not immune to similar criticism. Scientific neutrality in the field of psychotherapy is a myth. Luborsky et al. (1999) highlighted the 'researcher allegiance effect' whereby researchers show a marked tendency to find evidence that supports their therapeutic orientation (mostly cognitive and behavioural). From my own experience, I am aware of a striking antipathy in many of the scientists I have known to the sheer emotionality and irrationality of psychodynamic psychotherapy – an antipathy which unsurprisingly is in itself highly emotional and irrational.

My deepest concern is that the majority of children and adolescents who are presenting the greatest difficulties (and there are many, certainly more than current CAMHS can cope with) are being ill served by a kind of scientific prejudice that is threatening the very survival of psychodynamic therapeutic approaches in public services and the much needed help that they provide.

At the risk of being overly simplistic and reductionist, I think that it may well be the case that there are just two types of people who engage in scientific enquiry in the broad sense – those who learn at a distance through collecting and analysing data and those who learn 'close up' through direct emotional therapeutic involvement. The former may be frightened by the intensity of emotion in therapeutic work and take refuge in their relatively objective study. They may aspire to the greater precision and predictability of hard science (consumed with what has been called physics envy). The latter may be overly excited in their therapeutic involvement and may be simply unable to emerge sufficiently from their subjectivity.

They may seek something quite different, more imaginative and speculative maybe (which we might call, by comparison, poetry envy). Both types have their place in making sense of the mysteries of the psychotherapies. In the end, they look for different kinds of evidence to help them understand and improve their practice. What evidence works for whom?

References

American Psychiatric Association. *Diagnostic and Statistical Manual of Mental Health Disorders (DSM-5)*. Washington D.C.

CAMHS Evidence Based Practice Unit, University College, London. (2006). *Drawing on the Evidence; Advice for Mental Health Professionals Working With Children and Adolescents.*

CAMHS Evidence Based Practice Unit, University College and Anna Freud Centre (2007). *Choosing What's Best for You: What scientists have found helps children and young people who are sad, worried or troubled.* London: CAMHS Publications.

Fonagy, P. et al. (2002). *What Works for Whom? A Critical Review of Treatments for Children and Adolescents.* London: Guilford Press.

Guy, A. et al. (2011). *NICE under scrutiny; the Impact of the National Institute for Health and Clinical Excellence guidelines on the provision of psychotherapy in the UK.* London: UK Council for Psychotherapy.

IAPT (2010). *The IAPT Data Handbook: Guidance on recording and monitoring outcome to support local evidence-based practice,* IAPT National Program Team [Online]. Available: www.iapt.nhs.uk/services/measuring-outcomes (Accessed 20th December 2010). Appendices: www.iapt.nhs.uk/wp-content/uploads/iapt-data-handbook-appendices-v10.pdf.

Loewenthal, D. (ed.) (2015). *Critical Psychotherapy, Psychoanalysis and Counselling: Implications for Practice.* London: Palgrave Macmillan.

Loewenthal, D. and Samuels, A. (2014). *Relational Psychotherapy, Psychoanalysis and Counselling: Appraisal and reappraisal.* London: Routledge.

Luborsky, L. et al. (1999). The researcher's own therapy allegiances: A 'wild card' in comparisons of treatment efficacy. *Clinical Psychology: Science and Practice*, 6, 95–106.

Midgley, N. and Kennedy, E. (2011). Psychodynamic psychotherapy for children and adolescents: A critical review of the evidence base. *Journal of Child Psychotherapy*, 37 (3),1–29.

NICE (2004). *NHS Evidence – Defining Mental Health* [Online]. Available: www.library.nhs.uk/mentalhealth/viewresource.aspx?resid=105867 (Accessed 9th June 2010).

NICE (2009a). *Guideline Development Manual* [Online]. Available: www.nice. org.uk (Accessed 6th October 2010).

Rawlins, M.D. (2008). *De Testimonio. On the Evidence for Decisions about the use of Therapeutic interventions.* The Harveian Oration of 2008. Delivered for the Jack Tizard Memorial Lecture before the Fellows of The Royal College of Physicians of London on Thursday 16th October 2008, London: Royal College of Physicians. Slide notes available at https:// rcplondon.emea.acrobat.com/p37057603/ (Accessed 15th December 2010).

Shedler, J. (2010). The Efficacy of Psychodynamic Psychotherapy. *American Psychologist*, 65 (2), 98–109.

Thomas, P., Bracken, P. and Timimi, S. (2012). The Limits of Evidence–Based Medicine. *Philosophy, Psychiatry and Psychology*, 19 (4) 295–305.

Timimi, S. (2002). *Pathological Child Psychiatry and the Medicalisation of Childhood.* Hove: Brunner-Routledge.

Timimi, S. (2007). *Critical Voices in Child and Adolescent Mental Health.* London: Free Associations.

Timimi, S. (2013). No More Psychiatric Labels: Campaign to Abolish Psychiatric Diagnostic Systems such as ICD and DSM (CAPSID). *Self and Society*, 40 (4), 6–14.

Timimi, S. (2015). Children and young people's improving access to psychological therapies: Inspiring innovation or more of the same?. *BJP Bulletin*, 39, 57–60.

Weisz, J.R. (2014). Building Robust Psychotherapies for Children and Adolescents. *Perspectives on Psychological Science.*

Weisz, J.R. (2015, June). *MOD Squad for Youth Psychotherapy in Everyday Clinical Care: Transdiagnostic Treatment for Anxiety, Depression, and Conduct Problems.* (Delivered for the Jack Tizard Memorial Lecture before the Association for Child and Adolescent Mental Health, London).

World Health Organization. International Classification of Diseases, (ICD-10) (2004). Geneva: WHO.

YoungMinds (2015). *The Children's and Young People's Improving Access to Psychological Therapies Programme (CYP IAPT).* London: YoungMinds.

2

NON-DIAGNOSTIC PRACTICE IN CHILD AND ADOLESCENT MENTAL HEALTH

Sami Timimi

Diagnostic thinking has a powerful and pervasive impact on mental health services, structuring guidelines (such as the UK National Institute of Health and Care Excellence – NICE), research, administrative systems and care pathways. This chapter will examine the diagnosis-driven 'evidence base', which has become prescriptive for practice, not only in mental health, but also more widely across social care and education. Focusing on childhood psychiatric diagnoses such as attention-deficit/hyperactivity disorder (ADHD), autism and conduct disorder, the evidence base that supports (or otherwise) the scientific validity and clinical utility of using a diagnostic framework will be critically evaluated with particular reference to NICE guidelines. Ideas on how practice may develop in a direction that is effective, humane and more compatible with the scientific evidence will be outlined.

The problem with psychiatric diagnosis

For decades, concerned scientists and clinicians have called for a re-evaluation of the preeminent role of psychiatric diagnosis in organising and delivering mental health services. For example, in the United States, the Society for Humanistic Psychology's Global Summit on Diagnostic Alternatives (GSDA), a multidisciplinary group of researchers and practitioners, has brought together a wide range of institutions and individuals and is using

an Internet-based platform for furthering critique and propos-
ing change (http://dxsummit.org/). In the United Kingdom, the
British Psychological Society has produced a position paper calling for an end to using psychiatric diagnosis (Division of Clinical
Psychology of the British Psychological Society, 2013). Also in the
United Kingdom, a group of psychiatrists have written an influential position paper, now translated into several languages, pointing out that the evidence does not support the continued use
of the 'technical' model (matching treatments to diagnosis) and
instead recommends that, to be evidence based, services need to
move to 'relational' models of care (Bracken at al., 2012). For a
detailed review of the evidence on the lack of scientific basis or
clinical utility for psychiatric diagnosis, please see Timimi (2014a).
In brief the arguments against psychiatric diagnosis can be summarised as:

Psychiatric diagnoses are not valid

Unlike the rest of medicine, psychiatric diagnoses have failed to
connect their diagnoses with any causes. There are no physical tests
that can provide evidence for a diagnosis. Diagnoses in psychiatry
are descriptions of sets of behaviours that often go together. By itself
a psychiatric diagnosis cannot tell you about the cause, meaning
or best treatment. Even the descriptions of behaviours have large
crossovers between them. For example 'distractibility' can be found
in diagnoses such as ADHD, anxiety, depression and autism, as can
aggression, difficulties with making peer relationships and agita-
tion. This problem is predictable when the basis for the categories
is only 'symptoms' (behaviours) and not signs (measurable physical
differences). If, as now seems likely, our diagnoses do not reflect
real differences in our biology, then there is always a potential to
do harm if we use them as if they tell us something about the cause.
For example, if we believe that when a doctor makes a diagnosis of
ADHD they have discovered some real, possibly life-long, abnormality in that child's brain, we may accidentally lower everyone,
including that child's, expectation of what they can do and achieve,
at the same time as turning the focus on differences felt to be 'dys-
functional' and away from strengths and resources that the person
possesses.

Psychiatric diagnoses are not reliable

Reliability refers to the extent to which clinicians can agree on the same diagnoses when independently assessing a series of patients. No studies of diagnostic systems such as the American Diagnostic Statistical Manual (DSM), particularly when used in natural clinical settings, have shown high levels of reliability. Studies of reliability have found that reliability ratings in recent diagnostic manuals are not that different from those found in the 1970s. In DSM 5 (APA, 2013) field trials, the kappa coefficients (a statistical measure of agreement between two or more independent assessors), were uniformly poor with some common diagnoses such as major depressive disorder and generalised anxiety disorder achieving levels of inter-assessor agreement little better than chance.

Using psychiatric diagnosis does not aid treatment decisions

A positive outcome for treatment of psychiatric disorders is most strongly related to factors outside of treatment (such as social circumstances) and in treatment, the strongest association is with the strength of engagement with the treating clinician. Matching the diagnosis with a specific treatment (whether a specific drug or specific psychotherapy) has an insignificant effect.

Long-term prognosis for mental health problems has got worse

Unlike the rest of medicine, no overall improvement in mental health outcomes has been achieved in developed countries over the past half century. Some studies indicate that compared to a few decades ago there are more patients who have developed chronic conditions such as chronic schizophrenia than in the past. This is particularly so for young people, more of whom are being labelled as having a chronic (long-term) disability because of a mental condition than ever before, with rates of psychiatric medication being prescribed to children rising year on year without any accompanying evidence that their long-term outcomes are improving as a result.

Use of psychiatric diagnosis increases stigma

Surveys of public attitudes toward mental illness have found an increase in Western countries in the number of people who believe that mental illnesses are like other illnesses and caused by biological abnormalities such as a 'chemical imbalance' in the brain. However, the 'illness like any other illness' model is overwhelmingly associated with stigmatising attitudes such as a belief that patients are unpredictable and dangerous with associated fear of them and greater likelihood of wanting to avoid interacting with them.

Public health awareness campaigns have not improved outcomes

In order to increase rates of diagnosis and treatment of mental health problems, a variety of campaigns have been undertaken. These include the *'Defeat Depression'* campaign in the United Kingdom in the early 1990s that was intended to raise public awareness of depression, reduce stigma and improve rates of recognition and treatment. Another example is the *'Beyond Blue'* campaign in Australia, which has been running for over two decades and aims to increase awareness about depression and other mental health problems. Evaluations of both campaigns found no evidence that they led to any significant improvements in clinical outcomes, but were instead associated with a rapid increase in antidepressant and other psychoactive medication prescribing.

Psychiatric diagnosis imposes Western beliefs about mental distress on other cultures

Countries around the world are being encouraged to adopt Western beliefs and to recognise diagnoses like ADHD, schizophrenia and depression. However, outcomes, particularly for more severe mental conditions, have been consistently better in politically stable developing countries than developed ones. Several international studies have also concluded that the greater the inequality (in economic and social resources) in any society, the poorer the mental health. In the process of encouraging the adoption of Western psychiatric models, we not only imply that those cultures that are slow to take up these ideas are 'backward', but we may also undermine effective local practices and distract attention from factors that do make a difference to mental health such as economic ones.

Alternative evidence-based models for organising effective mental health care are available

We already know about many factors associated with greater likelihood of developing mental distress such as trauma, particularly early childhood trauma, adversity, socio-economic inequality, lifestyle and family functioning. In addition, rating levels of impairment and distress would provide a more accurate and less stigmatising way of categorising mental health problems than using psychiatric labels.

The message from research into outcomes from treatment of mental health problems is that using diagnostic categories to choose treatment models makes little difference, but concentrating on developing meaningful relationships with service users does. Service users, including young people, need to be included as active collaborators in their recovery. Furthermore, the biggest impact on outcomes comes from factors outside treatment such as social circumstances and levels of support. Evidence based services need therefore to learn how to work with the lived reality people experience, not just the space 'between the ears'. A more mature understanding of mental distress that is not based on wishful thinking or prejudice will recognise that mental health concerns us all. We can all suffer and we all have resources. Later in this chapter, I outline a model for developing services that incorporate this evidence into the delivery model.

National Institute of Health and Care Excellence (NICE) mental health guidelines

NICE guidelines in mental health are essentially 'eminence' based rather than 'evidence' based. That is, they are influenced more by 'who' was in the guideline group than what the evidence was pointing toward. In addition, because they are based on diagnostic concepts that are, as summarised above, not supportable scientifically or clinically, they fail to move treatment models in the direction of more effective and efficient care. I will illustrate these problematic issues by reference below to three NICE guidelines that, broadly speaking, try to encompass children's behaviour problems (see also Timimi, 2014b).

NICE guidelines on ADHD

The NICE Quick Reference Guide on ADHD doesn't mention any concern or controversy over the concept of ADHD. The full guideline (which few will read), however, has a more in-depth examination of validity (NICE, 2008). With each of the criterion, it takes a leap of faith to conclude that the available evidence supports the validity of the concept of ADHD. For example, on the question of whether ADHD can be distinguished from normal variation the full guideline concludes, '*Most analytic approaches are unable to make a clear distinction between the diagnosis of ADHD and the continuous distribution of ADHD symptoms in the general population*' (NICE, 2008: p104). On causal influences it notes that genetic factors have yet to be shown to be significantly associated with ADHD, '*As with all other types of risk factors associated with ADHD, the individual genetic variants associated with the disorder are neither sufficient nor necessary to cause it*' (NICE, 2008: p111). With neuroimaging studies, they note the lack of consistent findings. They also find some positive associations with a large number of familial and environmental adversity indicators. Little evidence is offered that any of the identified weak associated factors are specific to ADHD (as opposed to say conduct disorder) suggesting that if just about everything causes ADHD, then in fact we know nothing about what causes it.

NICE really departs from the evidence base when it comes to finding support for using stimulant medication as a first-line treatment in 'severe ADHD'. The review of pharmacotherapy studies notes the inadequate reporting of drug trial methodology, publication bias, limited reliability of results, inadequate data regarding adverse events and lack of evidence of long-term benefit, concluding that the evidence does not support using medication as a first-line treatment for 'mild or moderate' ADHD. However, it also concludes that medication should be offered as a first-line treatment in 'severe' ADHD with only one reference cited in support of this (Santosh et al., 2005), which concluded that in a 14-month randomised controlled trial, the more severe subgroup showed a larger decrease in symptoms from medication compared to behaviour therapy. Yet a 36-month follow up of the same patients could not find support for continuing beneficial effects of medication over behaviour therapy, regardless of initial severity (Swanson et al., 2007). Other naturalistic studies have come to similar conclusions finding that medication offers little prospect of improving long-term outcomes (Currie et al., 2013). It seems that a 'get out clause' that allows clinicians to categorise the problems as 'severe' was needed to enable existing practice to be maintained irrespective of what evidence was found. Five years after the publication of these guidelines, stimulant prescription in the United Kingdom had been raised by a further 56% from their already high levels at the time of publication (McClure, 2013).

NICE guidelines

With regard to autistic spectrum disorders (ASD), the NICE guideline encourages earlier recognition, which is likely to lead to a continuing increase in the numbers diagnosed with an ASD (Baird et al., 2011). This guideline did not consider evidence on the validity of the diagnosis, assuming its validity is a given. A diagnosis that is believed to be biologically driven and lifelong is at risk of causing significant harm through the negative impact of these assumptions on perceived competence, particularly if there are no objective findings to validate such a construct and no specific treatments available. The numbers are considerable as prevalence has expanded from 4 per 10,000 to 160 per 10,000 in just four decades – an increase of 3900% – but this impressive expansion has not come about through any new scientific discovery (Timimi et al., 2010).

Although it is assumed that ASD must be genetic, thus far molecular genetic studies including whole genome scans have found evidence for a non-significant proportion of the assumed total genetic risk with these small genetic associations being heterogeneous, crossing psychiatric diagnostic boundaries and more strongly related to learning difficulties than a diagnosis of ASD per se. Thus recent reviews of the genetic research in ASD published in *Nature* concluded, '*Many research teams have searched for genes that may be involved. They haven't turned up any prime candidates yet, only dozens, maybe hundreds of bit players*' (Hughes, 2012: S2) and '*Genome Wide Association Studies have failed to turn up any parts of the genome with statistical significance*' (Williams, 2012: S5).

Similarly autism neuroimaging studies have been plagued by heterogeneity issues resulting in a characteristic lack of consistently replicated findings with new theories regularly arriving and then departing. For example, studies focusing on the cerebellum have documented larger than average, smaller than average and no difference in cerebellar volume amongst children diagnosed with ASD compared to controls (Timimi et al., 2010).

There is also no evidence of methodologically sound and replicated research that demonstrates that particular interventions (whether educational, psychological, social or physical) specifically and differentially help those who have any form of autism (when compared to other children with behaviour or learning problems). Until specific treatments for ASD are adequately demonstrated through replicated controlled trials, we cannot and should not assume that the diagnosis has clinical value, at least in terms of treatment implications (Timimi et al., 2010).

With regard to prognosis, the same behaviourally defined syndrome (ASD) is applied to residents of institutions with little hope of living independently and has been suggested for men who have achieved greatness (such as Mozart, Van Gogh, Einstein, Edison and Darwin). From an 'impairment' perspective, this is virtually the entire human spectrum, suggesting ASD, as it is defined, is too heterogeneous to have prognostic value. Not surprisingly, recent prospective studies have shown remarkably diverse outcomes, with many who have been diagnosed with an ASD in childhood reportedly having few or no symptoms by adulthood (Szatmari, 2011).

NICE guidelines on conduct disorders

Having painstakingly tried to avoid the possibility that ADHD or ASD could be thought of as being connected with adverse environmental experiences, when it comes to conduct disorders (CD) the reverse is true. CD, we are told in the NICE summary guide, is associated with a greater likelihood of the child experiencing harsh and inconsistent parenting, parental mental health problems, environmental factors such as poverty and being looked after and individual factors such as low educational attainment and other mental health problems. The treatment recommendations thus focus on parent training programmes and other systemic interventions (NICE, 2013).

There is a worrying recommendation of using Risperidone off licence despite the poor evidence base for efficacy and the considerable health risks associated with it, but essentially we are left with no doubt that, unlike ADHD and ASD, CD is the result of poor environments. The solutions offered remain technical in nature, involving the usual tendency to give lip service to taking account of diversity, followed by recommending structured one-size-fits-all treatments (of particular parent training programmes).

Behaviour problems are not NICE compliant

Rather than reflecting the uncertainties present in ascribing behavioural issues in children to particular causes, the three NICE quick reference guides referred to above convey the false impression that children presenting with behaviour problems can be accurately categorised and from there a correct (and one-dimensional) process for stopping deviant behaviour can emerge. Sadly or gladly (depending on your perspective), in the real world children's behaviour does not emerge out of predictable algorithms that enable us to accurately identify separate features caused by genes, parents, teachers and so on, which then allow us to choose the 'correct' treatment. None of our medications treats a known biological abnormality and none has been shown to improve long-term outcomes.

Beyond diagnosis: How real-world services can become more effective

Mental health services are not always good for you. The figures on outcomes from treatment in real-world mental health settings in the developed world are nothing short of shocking. Lambert (2010) concluded that 75% of people entering community mental health centres in the United States are either not responding to treatment, or deteriorating while in care. Hansen and colleagues (2002), in a US study of over 6,000 mental health service users, reported a sobering picture of routine clinical care in which only 20% of clients improved. In Britain, the Centre for Social Justice (2012), reviewing the effectiveness data of a major project in National

Health mental health services, found only 15% of people entering the project were achieving 'recovery' by the time they left. In Australia, despite massive investment in mental health services in the past two decades, no corresponding improvement in the adult mental health of the population has been found (Jorm and Reavley, 2012).

A similar picture of poor outcomes in real-world child and adolescent mental health services has also been found. Weisz and colleagues (1995) reported that for traditional treatment in the community, the overall effect size of change for those attending community child and adolescent health services compared to those who weren't, was close to zero, a finding replicated in further studies (Weiss et al., 1999; 2000). Kazdin (2004) reported that 40–60% of youth who begin treatment drop out against advice, while Warren and colleagues (2009; 2010) found a deterioration rate of 24% amongst children in public community mental health settings.

Investigative medical journalist Robert Whitaker (2010) has documented a tripling of the number of disabled mentally ill in the United States over the past two decades. In 1955, there were around 350,000 adults in the US state and county mental systems with a psychiatric diagnosis, but the number categorised as disabled from mental illness rose to 4 million adults by 2007. Similarly, the numbers of youth in the United States categorised as having a disability because of a mental condition leapt from around 16,000 in 1987 to 560,000 in 2007. Whitaker suggests these increases could be a direct consequence of a parallel increase in the use of psychotropic drugs, which may have long-lasting and negative impacts on a person's ability to function (Whitaker, 2010).

The main message from outcome research is that diagnosis-driven models do not improve outcomes and services can improve outcomes by concentrating on developing meaningful relationships with service users that fully include them in decision-making processes (Bracken et al., 2012). Using flexible treatment models where there is regular testing through service user feedback of whether or not a particular intervention is improving outcomes for that service user has also been shown to improve outcomes and reduce the likelihood of becoming a 'long-term' patient (Duncan, 2014).

Partners for Change Outcome Management Systems (PCOMS)

One example of an approach that incorporates the evidence on what influences outcomes from treatment of mental health problems into a service delivery model is the Partners for Change Outcome Management Systems (PCOMS) project. PCOMS is a project developed in the United States that incorporates predictors of therapeutic success into an outcome-management system that includes simple, easy to use ratings of both therapeutic progress and alliance (Duncan, 2012; 2014). It moves the central task of therapeutic activity away from the primacy of the 'technical' (such as matching treatment to diagnosis) toward the primacy of the 'relational'. PCOMS has been shown in a number of randomised clinical trials to significantly improve effectiveness in clinical settings (Lambert and Shimokawa, 2011). Several agencies have conducted systematic analyses of real-life implementations of PCOMS (see Bohanske and Franczak, 2010; Reese et al., 2014) finding that non-attendance and length of time in treatment decrease, while outcomes for service users are closer in magnitude to that found in research than in other studies of real-life services such as those discussed above.

At the heart of the PCOMS approach is a non-diagnostic centred model of care incorporating systematic feedback of both outcome and alliance using non-symptom based brief measures. Therapeutic sessions start with the Outcome Rating Scale (ORS; Miller et al., 2003). The ORS is a visual analogue scale consisting of four 10 cm lines, corresponding to four domains (individual, interpersonal, social and overall). Patients, and/or their supporters, place a mark (or click a mouse in the online versions) on each line to represent their perception of their functioning in each domain. Practitioners measure each line (this is done automatically in online versions) to get a score out of 10 for each domain and a maximum score out of 40 once all four scores are added up. Lower scores reflect more distress. Graphing session by session scores enables patients and practitioners to notice whether or not positive change is being perceived by the patient, enabling conversations about change to take place. If change isn't happening practitioners can discuss with patients, their supporters and colleagues, what might be done differently such as a change of therapeutic modality, change in who attends the sessions or indeed a change in practitioner.

The Session Rating Scale (SRS; Duncan et al., 2003), also a four-item visual analogue scale, covers the traditional elements of the alliance, and is given toward the end of a therapeutic session. Each line on the SRS is 10 cm and can be scored manually or electronically. Using the SRS regularly inserts a ritual into therapy. This prompts practitioners to have a conversation with their patients about their experience of therapy. The SRS provides a structure to keep the alliance at the forefront of the practitioner's thinking, allowing an opportunity to fix any problems, and demonstrating that the therapist does more than lip service to the central task of forming good and empowering therapeutic relationships.

Systematic feedback models like PCOMS offer a more cost-effective and practical alternative as a quality improvement strategy compared to the transporting of evidence-based treatments in cumbersome diagnostic treatment matching strategies. Reese and colleagues (2014), for example, investigated the outcomes of 5,168 racially diverse, impoverished (below the US federal poverty level) adults who received therapy as part of a service that had implemented PCOMS in a public mental health setting. The overall effect sizes of treatment, regardless of diagnosis, were comparable to general research based outcomes and far superior to that found in mental health services in general. Diagnosis predicted neither the outcome nor length of stay in service.

Outcome Orientated Approaches to Mental Health Services (OO-AMHS)

A UK-based implementation of the PCOMS approach – Outcome Orientated Approaches to Mental Health (OO-AMHS) (Timimi et al., 2013) – has also found similar positive outcomes following implementation in a child and adolescent mental health service (CAMHS). Implementing OO-AMHS in a community CAMHS in Lincolnshire in the United Kingdom moved practice away from a focus on diagnostic based 'symptom management' paradigms and toward collaborative, patient and family empowering model of care, with treatments building on the primacy of relational aspects of care in preference to the primacy of technical ones.

OO-AMHS is a whole service transformation model that promotes recovery and person-centred care and embeds values such as promoting hope, noticing strengths, empowering patient voice and choice, respecting diversity, promoting social justice across the team and in service delivery with patients. The four CORE components of the OO-AMHS model are:

➤ **Consultation:** Prompt collaboration with other agencies ensures only services likely to promote a positive change engage with treatment,

➤ **Outcomes:** Obtaining ongoing, session-by-session patient-rated outcome data, using the ultra-brief 'Outcome Rating Scale' (ORS – discussed above), and changing treatment if outcomes are not improving,

➤ **Relationships:** Developing effective therapeutic alliances aided by the patient-rated experience ultra-brief tool – the Session Rating Scale (SRS – discussed above),

➤ **Ethics of care:** Developing positive and caring team cultures that are recovery focused and understand how to use outcome data for clinical reflection, supervision, and whole-team development.

The OO-AMHS model, building on the PCOMS approach, benefits from high feasibility and requires minimal training. Unlike other service transformation projects, there is no requirement to train clinicians in evidence-based treatments. Instead implementation involves helping clinicians maximise effective use of already existing skills by team development, working more productively with other agencies and by using the feedback tools ORS and SRS to quickly identify patients who are not progressing, or where the alliance has issues, and changing the approach taken with them.

Evidence from implementation of the OO-AMHS approach within a community CAMHS in Lincolnshire found, after nearly two years of implementation, that the number of cases with the service for over two years had reduced from 38% of the caseload to 18%, numbers referred for in-patient treatment had also come down from 15 per year to 3 per year, and non-attendance rates had dropped significantly. Analysis of over 300 cases discharged from this team post implementation found 77% of those discharged had shown clinically significant improvement and/or were above the clinical cut-off (recovered), with only 6% rating deterioration in their condition.

Conclusion

In this chapter, I have argued that psychiatric diagnosis does not provide a rational basis for organising and delivering mental health services. Thus, it is not surprising that studies of outcomes achieved by real-world mental health services show such a poor record. I also argued that effective alternatives already exist, with evidence that they can improve the outcomes delivered by real-world psychiatric services, and the approach developed in the United States known as the 'Partners for Change Outcome Management Systems' (PCOMS) and a UK derivative 'Outcome Orientated Approaches to Mental Health Services' (OO-AMHS). Effective, evidence-based and human alternatives to the current narrow, largely bio-medical and/or technical models exist and would be relatively straightforward to scale up. The political challenge for us all is an implementation rather than evidence-based one.

References

American Psychiatric Association (2013). *Diagnostic and Statistical Manual of Mental Disorders Fifth Edition (DSM 5)*. Washington D.C.: American Psychiatric Association.

Baird, G., Douglas, H.R. and Murphy, S. (2011). Recognising and diagnosing autism in children and young people with autism; summary of the NICE guidelines: The matrix of assessment and treatment of autism spectrum disorders. *British Medical Journal, 343*, d6360.

Bohanske, R.T. and Franczak, M. (2010). Transforming public behavioral health care: A case example of consumer-directed services, recovery, and the common factors. In B.L. Duncan, S.D. Miller, B.E. Wampold and M.A. Hubble (eds), *The Heart and Soul of Change, 2nd Edition: Delivering What Works in Therapy*. Washington: American Psychological Association.

Bracken, P., Thomas, P., Timimi, S. et al. (2012). Psychiatry beyond the current paradigm. *British Journal of Psychiatry, 201*, 430–434.

Centre for Social Justice (2012). *Commissioning effective talking therapies*. Available at www.centreforsocialjustice.org.uk/publications/commissioning-effective-talking-therapies (Accessed 28th July 2015).

Currie, J., Stabile, M. and Jones, L.E. (2013). *Do Stimulant Medications Improve Educational and Behavioral Outcomes for Children with ADHD? NBER Working Paper No. 19105*. Cambridge, MA: National Bureau of Economic Research.

Division of Clinical Psychology of the British Psychological Society (2013). *Division of Clinical Psychology Position Statement on the classification of behaviour and experience in relation to functional psychiatric diagnoses: Time for a paradigm shift.* Available at www.madinamerica.com/wp-content/uploads/2013/05/DCP-Position-Statement-on-Classification.pdf (Accessed 28th July 2015).

Duncan, B. (2012). The partners for change outcome management system (PCOMS): The heart and soul of change project. *Canadian Psychology*, 53, 93–104.

Duncan, B. (2014). *On becoming a better therapist: Evidence based practice one client at a time (2nd edition).* Washington, DC: American Psychological Association.

Duncan, B., Miller, S., Sparks, J., Claud, D., Reynolds, L. and Brown, J. (2003). The Session Rating Scale: Preliminary psychometric properties of a 'working' alliance measure. *Journal of Brief Therapy*, 3, 3–12.

Hansen, N., Lambert, M. and Forman, E. (2002). The psychotherapy dose-effect and its implications for treatment delivery services. *Clinical Psychology: Science and Practice*, 9, 329–343.

Hughes, V. (2012). A complex disorder, *Nature*, 491, 7422, S2.

Jorm, A.F. and Reavley, N.J. (2012). Changes in psychological distress in Australian adults between 1995 and 2011. *Australian and New Zealand Journal of Psychiatry*, 46, 352–356.

Kazdin, A.E. (2004). Psychotherapy for children and adolescents. In M.J. Lambert (ed.), *Bergin and Garfield's Handbook of Psychotherapy and Behavior Change.* New York: Wiley.

Lambert, M.J. (2010). *Prevention of treatment failure: The use of measuring, monitoring, and feedback in clinical practice.* Washington, DC: APA Press.

Lambert, M.J. and Shimokawa, K. (2011). Collecting client feedback. *Psychotherapy*, 48, 72–79.

McClure, I. (2013). Prescribing methylphenidate for moderate ADHD. *British Medical Journal*, 347, f6216

Miller, S.D., Duncan, B.L., Brown, J., Sparks, J. and Claude, D. (2003). The outcome rating scale: A preliminary study of the reliability, validity, and feasibility of a brief visual analog measure. *Journal of Brief Therapy*, 2, 91–100.

National Institute for health and Care Excellence (NICE) (2008). *Attention Deficit Hyperactivity Disorder: Diagnosis and management of ADHD in children, young people and adults. National Clinical Practice Guideline Number 72.* London: NICE.

National Institute for health and Clinical Excellence (NICE) (2013). *Antisocial Behaviour and Conduct Disorders in Children and Young People. National Clinical Guideline Number 158.* Leicester: British Psychological Society and London: Royal College of Psychiatrists.

Reese, R.J., Duncan, B., Bohanske, R., Owen, J. and Minami, T. (2014) Benchmarking outcomes in a public behavioral health setting: Feedback as a quality improvement strategy. *Journal of Consulting and Clinical Psychology*, 82, 731–742.

Santosh, P., Taylor, E., Swanson, J. et al. (2005). Refining the diagnoses of inattention and overactivity syndromes: A reanalysis of the Multimodal Treatment study of attention deficit hyperactivity disorder (ADHD) based on ICD-10 criteria for hyperkinetic disorder. *Clinical Neuroscience Research*, 5, 307–14.

Swanson, J.M., Hinshaw, S.P., Arnold L.E. et al. (2007). Secondary evaluations of MTA 36-month outcomes: propensity score and growth mixture model analyses. *Journal of the American Academy of Child and Adolescent Psychiatry*, 46, 1003–1014.

Szatmari, P. (2011). New recommendations on autism spectrum disorder. *British Medical Journal*, 342, d2456.

Timimi, S. (2014a). No More Psychiatric Labels: Why formal psychiatric diagnostic systems should be abolished. *International Journal of Clinical and Health Psychology*, 14, 208–215.

Timimi, S. (2014b). Children's behaviour problems: A NICE mess. *International Journal of Clinical Practice*, 68, 1053–1055.

Timimi, S., Tetley, D., Burgoine, W. and Walker, G. (2013). Outcome Orientated Child and Adolescent Mental Health Services (OO-CAMHS): A whole service model. *Clinical Child Psychology and Psychiatry*, 18, 169–184.

Timimi, S., McCabe, B. and Gardner, N. (2010). *The Myth of Autism: Medicalising Boys' and Men's Social and Emotional Competence*. Basingstoke: Palgrave Macmillan.

Warren, J.S., Nelson, P.L. and Burlingame, G.M. (2009). Identifying youth at risk for treatment failure in outpatient community mental health services. *Journal of Child and Family Studies*, 18, 690–701.

Warren, J.S., Nelson, P.L., Mondragon, S.A., Baldwin, S.A. and Burlingame, G.M. (2010). Youth psychotherapy change trajectories and outcomes in usual care: Community mental health versus managed care settings. *Journal of Consulting and Clinical Psychology*, 78, 144–155.

Weiss, B., Catron, T. and Harris, V. (1999). The effectiveness of traditional child psychotherapy. *Journal of Consulting and Clinical Psychology*, 67, 82–94.

Weiss, B., Catron, T. and Harris, V. (2000). A two-year follow-up of the effectiveness of traditional child psychotherapy. *Journal of Consulting and Clinical Psychology*, 68, 1094–1101.

Weisz, J.R., Donenberg, G.R. and Weiss, B. (1995). Bridging the gap between laboratory and clinic in child and adolescent psychotherapy: efficacy and effectiveness in studies of child and adolescent psychotherapy *Journal of Consulting and Clinical Psychology*, 63, 688–701.

Whitaker, R. (2010). *Anatomy of an Epidemic*. New York: Crown.

Williams, S.C. (2012). Searching for answers. *Nature*, 491, 7422, S4–S6.

3

NEUROSCIENCE AND CAMHS PRACTICE

Matthew Woolgar and Carmen Pinto

Introduction

On television, a popular scientist explains that the implications on a child of the impact of witnessing domestic violence are deep and profound; they tap the side of their skull to emphasise just how deep within the child's brain the legacy of this must reside and how difficult it will therefore be to access and change. At a professionals' meeting, a teenage girl with a history of challenging behaviour is considered a hopeless case because of all that she has suffered early on in life and now there is little left that anyone can do to reach deep inside her mind and turn her around. The legacy of her abuse has changed her brain. A mother cries outside a child and adolescent mental health services (CAMHS) clinic having been told that her postnatal depression meant that she failed to nurture her infant's brain at the critical time point and it is now this that explains her son's ADHD and reading problems.

There is no doubt that early experiences can be very important for later development and that science is unpacking some of the ways that neglect and maltreatment can affect various biological systems. Our concern in this chapter is not at all with questioning the usefulness of the biological sciences, which we believe greatly enhance our understanding of cases, and especially complex ones, but more to reflect on some of the science and the extent to which it is ready to make the journey into everyday practice settings in a reliable way. And our main concern relates to the risks of overstating a too simplistic neuroscience conceptualisation. We offer a suggestion to go back to a personalised biopsychosocial formulation to ensure all the factors are considered and argue that the broader science urges us to think about individual differences and in particular of differential susceptibility.

Example of overstating the case of neuroscience

The question has to be the extent to which this new brain science is able to inform our understanding of specific cases in CAMHS. There are papers and reviews which discuss the complexity of the science (Woolgar, 2013) as well as some of the possible social risks (Edwards et al., in press). The first thing to consider is how well such a technical science can be understood and translated into practical settings. Neuroscientists themselves have commented on the difficulty of translating their findings into public discourse. In a review conducted by Harvard University into the public presentation of the emerging neuroscience, it was noted that 'the substantive content of the science was often misinterpreted or misrepresented' (Shonkoff and Bales, 2011: 18). This review has led to an online project to increase public understanding with the creation of the centre for the Developing Child at Harvard University (www.youtube.com/user/HarvardCenter), which includes short videos explaining key concepts in everyday language such as the transactional nature of the mechanism by which experience shapes brain development, for example in terms of 'serve and return'. But it is not just the public understanding that needs to be addressed. Leading neuroscientists have also said:

> ... the chronicling of links between parenting and brain structure and function... is no more important, from the perspective of either basic or applied science, than documenting such links between parenting and children's development more generally. As it turns out, the study of parenting and brain development is not even yet in its infancy; it would be more appropriate to conclude that it is still in the embryonic stage, if not that which precedes conception... (Belsky and de Haan, 2011: 409)

The science is opening up new avenues of understanding but it is not yet the case that these are more valuable than our traditional approaches to understanding complex child behaviour.

These concerns from neuroscientists are evidenced by the extent to which 'neuromyths' have taken hold (Howard-Jones, 2014). This paper presented a study that showed the prevalence of such neuromyths in educational settings, and how they have been used to attempt to influence teaching programmes in a supposedly evidence-informed way. These neuromyths sounded very believable at face value, and included statements such as 'We mostly only use 10% of our brain' and 'Short bouts of co-ordination exercise can improve the integration of left and right hemispheric brain function' which were believed by 48% and 88% respectively of teachers sampled in the United Kingdom and at similar rates in teachers across the Netherlands, Turkey, Greece and China. The paper also highlighted the pervasiveness of 'The Myth of Three' which in education has been driven by the Heckman model (see Figure 3.1), which appears to show, as an established fact, based on neuroscientific evidence, the economic benefit of investing in early education, especially pre-school education, in terms of giving tax-payers more power per pound invested.

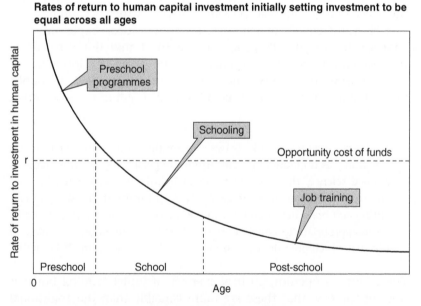

Figure 3.1 The Heckman model (Heckman, 2008)

The author notes that 'this simple model considerably detracts from our modern understanding of the brain' (p. 820) because it is based on several tenuous and outdated assumptions that do not reflect current understanding of the fluidity and complexity of brain development. Importantly, this graph is not based on empirical data at all, despite what it might look like, but is a theory based only on some assumptions. When empirical data relevant to this theory have been plotted, whilst they do indeed show some benefits for early intervention, the model is complex and these effects are especially true for more disadvantaged children. Nonetheless, the Myth of Three has been largely uncritically absorbed into CAMHS provision as well, with an emphasis on early intervention as the most effective use of funds.[1]

Having said this, there is an abundance of evidence that demonstrates the consequences for brain development and functioning that follows from neglect, maltreatment and abuse (McCrory et al., 2010). But again simplistic explanations are not helpful. One of the most common images used to illustrate the impact on neurodevelopment of maltreatment is a brain scan image of a normal three-year-old brain and an extremely neglected three-year-old brain side by side. Many safeguarding trainings in CAMHS now frequently use this image and of course it has appeared on the front of the cross-party review on the importance of early intervention (http://media.education.gov.uk/assets/files/pdf/g/graham%20 allens%20review%20of%20early%20intervention.pdf).   However it has also been described as possibly the most misleading image in neuroscience (The Big Think: http://bigthink.com/neurobonk-ers/is-this-the-most-misleading-image-in-neuroscience).   Whatever else one might think about this image, and there are a number of criticisms that people have made about it over the years, not least the absence of a shared scale, it is probably wise to consider it unhelpful for shaping and determining policy in general and certainly for individual children's experiences. The differences between the normal brain and the composite of neglected children's brain are so extreme they are unlikely to reflect useful real-life experience. You are very unlikely to see a difference so marked, in terms of head circumference, for any neglected child you might ever meet. If we assume these images are on the same scale, then taken at face value, because the normal one is described as being on the 50th percentile for a three-year-old, the neglected brain of the three-year-old on the right appears to be about the size of a neonate, and that is exceptionally unlikely based what we know about head circumferences (www.who.int/childgrowth/standards/second_set/chts_hcfa_boys_p/en/).

Maltreatment and neurodevelopment

In this next section we review some of the literature relevant to the neurodevelopmental legacy of early maltreatment and neglect. The brain can respond to non-optimal environments in terms of both its structure and architecture, that is, the way it looks on brain scans, or in terms of its function, which relates to how it works, or more specifically the pattern of activity seen in different regions when it is doing its work of thinking. In terms of changes in structure measured through scans such as CT or MRI scans one gets a static picture of the areas of the brain that may be larger or denser compared to those in other brains which are smaller or more hollowed out. But perhaps more interesting are the scans that look at the functional differences in terms of how the brain does its thinking, how efficiently it does the thinking and in what parts of the brain that thinking takes place. This dynamic information of the brain at work can be gleaned from a variety of sources such as functional MRI (or f-MRI) scanning as well as event-related potential studies using EEG systems (typically measured with a participant wearing a net on their head, and the changes in the electrical activity beneath the skull picked up by carefully placed sensors on the net).

An example of the use of a structural MRI scanning study is one which looked at the differences in size, or volume of parts of the brain, in a population of female undergraduates who reported sexual abuse occurring at different stages of their life (Andersen et al., 2008). The aim of this study was to test the hypothesis that different parts of the brain are developmentally susceptible to specific environmental stresses at different ages. In this instance childhood sexual abuse in young women was associated with reductions in the volume of the hippocampus region when the abuse occurred early on in life (between two time periods 3 to 5 years and 11 to 13 years), whilst the corpus callosum was affected when sexual abuse had occurred during the ages of 9 to 10 years and the frontal cortex in older children aged between 14 and 16 years. Importantly, these time-limited effects are broadly consistent with the periods within which those parts of the brain normally show the greatest development and thus it is suggested that the stress that occurred secondary to childhood sexual abuse in these women's childhoods was having a differential impact on those stages of the brain which were differentially developing during that period. This makes a lot of sense from the point of view of developmental science, which has demonstrated specific periods in the brain's development, and the susceptibility of these regions to forms of environmental insult – at least in this sample of young women during their growing up. How this important research translates directly into the clinic is not entirely clear. But it may serve to highlight the idea that sexual abuse at different points in life may have different consequences for the victim, which makes sense, but note that in this study no association was reported between these changes in brain volumes and any associated outcomes in young adulthood of this sample of college women. What was seen in the scanner did not predict how these young women were functioning. The ability to map these discrete brain changes to different patterns of psychopathology or wellbeing would be extremely interesting but without that it may simply serve to remind us that childhood sexual abuse can have a variety of impacts on its victim as we know from pre-existing research already (Widom, 2012).

An example of the more dynamic types of assessment permitted by f-MRI scans is derived from a series of studies by Pollak and colleagues (Pollak, 2008), which have shown that maltreated children have specific biases towards identifying angry emotions, but not other emotions, in emotionally ambiguous faces. This has been revealed by increases in brain activity (processing) when being vigilant for, orienting towards and then delaying their look away from specifically angry faces. Later studies showed that these effects were not just within the brain but also extended into physiological measures such as skin conductance and heart rate, highlighting the importance of looking beyond just the brain to see the broader biological legacy of early environments (see below). These changes in brain functioning were seemingly associated with an acquired hypervigilance towards angry sources of emotion and the environment and would suggest some kind of adaptation towards living in a hostile environment. This raises the important point that changes in brain functioning associated with maltreatment and neglect may not be best thought of simply as damage done to the child, but rather as adaptations to a non-optimal environment. There is evidence from other neurobiological correlates of maltreatment and abuse that some of what looks like damage is in fact a more or less appropriate coping response to being in a difficult environment. Thus it makes sense for a maltreated child to be on the watch for angry faces in particular as these may indicate a potential threat in their environment of impending significant harm, which needs to be avoided. The problem comes of course when, or if, the environment undergoes a significant change, for example if maltreated children are moved from a hostile environment into a safer one and they may retain these preconscious biases towards seeking out threatening signals in their environment. For example, they may misinterpret the nurturing overtures of foster carers or adoptive parents towards them and so respond in non-adaptive ways, at least whilst such neurological biases remain. This introduces the concept of plasticity and the possibility for change.

The idea that the brain changes and responds to variations in the prevailing environment is often referred to as its plasticity. It is a very important construct that is often helpfully contrasted with the idea of the importance of early sensitive periods for shaping the foundations of brain development and then of the brain as a static organ after these first few years. It is an important idea, but some neuroscientists argue that the notion of plasticity is itself problematic because the brain undergoes changes in its structure and function all the time – else how would we learn? – and that the understanding of this term is so wide and varied that it is not terribly helpful (Ariel-Shaw and McEachern, 2001). There are no doubt structural changes in the brain when we learn things, as has been demonstrated by the effects of learning to juggle or of London taxi drivers acquiring 'the Knowledge' (Draganski et al., 2004; Woollett and Maguire, 2011). But what most people typically mean when they use the term plasticity is at the functional level in which higher order skills are either recovered when they have been lost, say following a stroke or brain injury, and become relocated or picked up by other parts of the brain. But such gross damage in brain structure or function and then clear recovery is not usually characteristic of the consequences of maltreatment or neglect. But we know that change can happen in the biological legacy of maltreatment and neglect – that children who have experienced very difficult starts can adapt to new environments (Fisher et al., 2007;

Dozier et al., 2008) but we also know that this capacity differs from child to child. This introduces the sense of personalisation of effects and the idea of differential susceptibility.

Personalisation and individuals

We have seen how the timing of maltreatment, in terms of child-hood sexual abuse in young women, can have different structural impacts upon the development of the brain. We have also seen how exposure to maltreatment can lead to cortical level biases towards angry faces specifically, but that there are also biological legacies beyond the brain in terms of a child's physiology as well. We are not going to address it here but it has also been shown that maltreatment can have an impact not just on neurodevelopment and physiology but also on immunology and very importantly upon a child's genetics. Given that there are so many potential domains influenced in different ways and at different times in a child's life, and that different children appear to show different responses to changes in their environment, then we need to take into account the wide range and plurality of possible outcomes when a child is subjected to maltreatment. In other words, we need to avoid thinking in terms of the scientific evidence pointing towards gross, reliable and possibly inevitable difficulties at the biological level subsequent to maltreatment and neglect and think more about the individual child's specific formulation, because this is what the broader science does in fact lead us towards.

In fact the science is very clear that there are individual, biological reasons why different children would be likely to show different responses and outcomes to similar types of maltreatment, even if that maltreatment were to operate at the same point in their lives. One of the best models for explaining this is differential susceptibility (Belsky, Bakermans-Kranenburg and van IJzendoorn, 2007). A model that is largely understood in terms of genetics but which can be thought of as to do with many things within the child more generally, not least because genes and environments start to mutually shape and transact with each other from the moment of conception and therefore to disentangle the effects of one from the other becomes rather complicated (van IJzendoorn, Bakermans-Kranenburg and Ebstein, 2011).

It has long been known that some individuals are more susceptible to risk environments than others (the stress-diathesis model) but there is increasing evidence for outcomes, including behaviour problems, depression and even attachment disorganisation that the susceptibility can go both ways. Whilst some children may be especially vulnerable to relatively low levels of toxic environments, they may also, for similar reasons, be more responsive to improvements in their environments than other children. In this conceptualisation, the positive resource of 'resilience' is described in terms of being 'fixed', that is, relatively invariant according to the environmental conditions. The susceptible children are very sensitive to variations in their environment, so that they may suffer terribly in a negative environment, but flourish in a positive environment that is tailored exactly to their needs – and indeed may end up with higher quality outcomes than resilient children offered an equally positive environment. A metaphor that has been used to describe this phenomenon is a Swedish phrase about orchids and dandelions; children who are especially context sensitive are orchids who need very specific conditions to thrive, whilst those who grow at their own level whatever the context (i.e. are resilient) are the dandelions (Boyce and Ellis, 2005). These individual differences to the response to risk, which exist at the biological level, are important for thinking about a range of outcomes for children exposed to non-optimal environments and help us think about the biopsychosocial formulation for any particular child.

Biological prenatal influences on child development

A commonly understood way in which the environment can have a negative impact on brain development is the exposure to toxins in the womb. If we consider some of the toxins that an embryo can be exposed to in the womb, we can see how there is not a straightforward relationship between the toxin and the child's developmental outcomes. There are likely to be individual differences to exposure and some foetuses are likely to be more differentially susceptible, and indeed the causes of some difficulties may be much more complex than they seem at first, even beyond the direct exposure to the toxin. So again we must consider the actual child in front of us, rather than assume that we already know about the biological damage done. Here we very briefly consider some of the research relating to the neurodevelopmental outcomes associated with three common toxins associated with maternal lifestyle during pregnancy; smoking, cocaine use and alcohol, which frequently appear in the developmental histories of children exposed to maltreatment and neglect.

Firstly, it is widely known that exposure to alcohol in the womb can have a negative effect on the unborn child, potentially leading to foetal alcohol-related disorders (e.g., foetal alcohol disorder, FAD) and a spectrum of less severe outcomes, encompassing growth retardation (height and/or weight) facial features and the rather diffuse idea of involvement of the central nervous system, which could be some combination of structural, neurological or functional (Barrow and Riley, 2011). However, the impact of alcohol is not straightforwardly related to the amount of exposure. This is why government warnings of the 'safe' amount to consume in pregnancy vary. No amount is truly safe because the susceptibility to alcohol depends on a number of factors, including the genetics of both the foetus and the mother. Indeed the spectrum of difficulties associated with alcohol exposure are also probably related to the differential susceptibility across different domains of functioning that each foetus has, and indeed to the differential capacity of the mother to metabolise alcohol and its products effectively (Tunc-Ozcan et al., 2014). Hence the inconsistency over the years as to what the safe level of alcohol during pregnancy is, not least because the most critical period for alcohol exposure for FAD is thought to be the first trimester, a time in which not all mothers-to-be are aware they are pregnant. As such some may be made to feel guilty if they have unwittingly 'exposed' their foetus to even small albeit, on the balance of probabilities, likely safe amounts of alcohol. But if a foetus (and/or the mother) are differentially susceptible to the effects of alcohol, then no amount can be said with certainty to be truly safe, and as we do not know how to predict this susceptibility many campaigners now promote a zero-tolerance based on the theory that there may be a significant risk with even a very small amount for some people. But unfortunately even if this risk truly exists, we do not know its magnitude nor how many would be affected. But beyond the case of health promotion, we also need to be careful about attributing a child's current presentation to a history of alcohol exposure in utero – other biopsychosocial factors often go alongside alcohol exposure in pregnancy, including parental mental health and neurodevelopmental factors. Furthermore, the likelihood that various genetic risks are likely to be more or less susceptible to the effect of alcohol means that a child whose development has been affected by in utero alcohol exposure may present in many different ways. These need to be considered on a case-by-case basis, and consideration given to the possibility that some of the presentation may be due to in utero exposure and some due to factors unrelated to alcohol exposure.

Smoking in pregnancy is well known to be associated with a range of negative child outcomes. The biological effects, in part to do with the reduction of oxygen to the foetus secondary to the nicotine, have been associated with lower birth weight, prematurity, sudden infant death syndrome, congenital malformations and differences in organ and brain functioning (Pickett and Wakschlag, 2011). But some research has suggested that the specific effects on child IQ and later school attainment that have been described in several studies may be less to do with the environmental exposure to smoking and more to do with the shared genes between a mother who smokes and her baby (D'Onofrio et al., 2010). That is, that women who smoke in pregnancy tend to have lower IQs than women who do not and the highly heritable trait of IQ is passed on to shape the child's cognitive functioning. So sometimes what seems certain to be an obvious environmental cause, with a seemingly biological mechanism, may only be an indicator of something else altogether, that is harder to quantify and in this case the smoking may be an indicator of lower maternal IQ rather than its primary biological cause. Nonetheless, the other negative effects of smoking, for example, on birth weight, remain more directly associated with the biological exposure itself.

Finally, children who have been born to substance misusing mothers are rightly of major concern for health services and a history of in utero substance abuse is common in many developmental histories of children in care. But the impact does depend on the type of substance misused. For example, despite the strength of the drug, there are relatively small effects reliably found for exposure to cocaine misuse (Singer and Minnes, 2011), and for those that have been found (post-natal growth; language; neurodevelopmental features) there is evidence that factors associated with the cocaine misusing lifestyle – for example, malnutrition, exposure to environmental toxins such as lead and possibly the post-natal parenting quality – may be more influential than the direct physiological impact of the drug itself (Singer et al., 2008; Ackerman et al., 2010). Thus in this instance the drug use may be an indicator of broader environmental risk factors associated with an impoverished maternal lifestyle rather than a direct effect of chemical toxicity.

So, alcohol effects are probably influenced by the genetic susceptibility of the mother/foetus, and indeed the outcomes (the behavioural phenotype) can be quite diverse and so the risk of and presentation due to the impact of prenatal alcohol exposure will vary from dyad to dyad. For smoking, some, but not all, of the negative outcomes may be related to the mother's pre-existing genetics rather than to her smoking. And for cocaine use, the broader lifestyle factors and especially the poorer-quality rearing environments may be a clearer explanatory factor than the drug's toxicity itself. This very brief overview hopefully conveys that the knowledge of the biological science leads to a range of possible outcomes and different mechanisms and as such a lot of unknowns for the individual child. In the absence of certainty, even biological certainty, it is better to have hypotheses about the individual child to guide our formulations that include the biology alongside the social and psychological factors.

Biopsychosocial model and formulation for personalised care in complex cases

A clinical formulation provides a hypothetical explanation of a child's presentation at a given time based on scientific and clinical knowledge. It relates the theoretical knowledge to practice and provides a plausible account of why the child seems to behave the way they do (Butler, 1998; Kuyken et al., 2009). The clinician doing the formulation has to take into account information from different sources, at different points in time, and in different domains, and link them with the specific child's thoughts, feelings and behaviours. A clinical formulation uses theory to make explanatory inferences about causes, triggering and maintaining factors that can inform interventions.

The biopsychosocial formulation involves considering a range of relevant biological, psychosocial and contextual factors. So, to make sense of the most complex cases in particular, the clinician needs to have expertise in the latest scientific evidence that informs conceptual and explanatory frameworks (genetics, social learning theory, cognitive-behavioural, systemic, etc.).

Formulation also includes a chronological aspect (Macneil et al., 2012), thinking about how issues have developed over time, beginning with historical predisposing factors that we know from the literature can potentially trigger a specific outcome (e.g. maternal alcohol use and a range of neurodevelopmental problems) in some people. Then the factors precipitating or triggering the current episode are identified and these are going to be specific to that child. Even though we know from research what common triggering factors are (e.g. changing school, family life event, bullying, etc.), not all children respond equally to the same life events and opportunities. Likewise, the formulation can also hypothesise what factors may perpetuate the problem if they remain unaltered, for example as research has found, children with untreated ADHD keep on doing poorly academically if their problems are not treated effectively (Scheffler et al., 2009). And last, but not least, formulation includes what resilience elements may help the child in their present and future functioning.

It is important to highlight that formulation offers a hypothesis about the causes and nature of the presenting problems and also provides a framework for developing the most suitable treatment approaches. It remains a hypothesis because some of the factors are common to large numbers of people, but they may not precisely apply to that particular child. So this links to the uncertainty about the natural history of a problem, and with the fact that each child needs to be understood as an individual. In contrast, diagnosis identifies what is common and predictable in the child's presentation whilst formulation considers what is unique and variable (Mace and Binyon, 2005). Both formulation and diagnosis help clinicians to devise a specifically-tailored treatment plan, but formulation helps to keep the child's uniqueness in mind and an openness to new explanations: exactly what we need to be able to integrate the emerging biological sciences, including neuroscience, into CAMHS practice.

Case study Box 3.1

Calliope is a 13-year-old looked-after girl who was referred to a specialist adoption and fostering mental health service by social services. Her social worker was concerned that she was suffering from 'an attachment disorder and neurodevelopmental trauma due to neglect and abuse' but no account was provided in the referral as to what this looked like (i.e. how it presented in her) and why this might be – it seemed to be based solely on her history of being in care. There are no obvious treatments or care pathways for such a vague description.

Calliope was removed from her mother's house when she was six years old, after witnessing domestic violence and experiencing physical abuse. She was always late for school, usually dirty and hungry. She was placed in foster care, and this soon broke down due to behavioural problems. Then she moved from two further brief placements due to similar problems and finally she achieved stability with her current foster carer. When she was assessed, she had been with her fourth foster carer, who was very experienced, for two years.

Her history revealed that her birth mother did not finish education, despite being described as bright, and since then she had not held down a job. Her mother was described as always rushing things and found tasks like learning or reading 'impossible' because her mind would wander off. Two of Calliope's birth siblings, now adopted, had a diagnosis of ADHD, as well as some of her cousins. It was thought that her mother took drugs and alcohol during pregnancy.

A multidisciplinary assessment involving clinical interviews with her foster carer, school and Calliope was conducted. A school observation also followed to clarify some of the issues. The foster carer described severe behavioural problems present when she first moved in, which after a while improved, but had now come back: Calliope was described as very oppositional, refusing to do as she was told, frequently arguing with adults and doing things to annoy the other foster children. Her foster carer was particularly worried about Calliope lying to get what she wanted, and the physical aggression towards her and the other children. She had punched, hit, kicked and pulled hair, and on a few occasions, she had used a pen as a weapon, stabbing her foster carer. This behaviour extended to school, where she tended to initiate physical fights and disturb the lessons. She had numerous detentions and was on the verge of permanent exclusion. In the assessment Calliope was equally non-compliant with the assessor, being rude and defiant.

When asked about her usual levels of attention and concentration, her foster carer described these as 'non-existent'. She could not focus for even five minutes on reading and always avoided homework, or any activity that required mental effort. She could not even take her to the cinema, as she would become bored long before the end of the film. Her foster carer described how Calliope was always fidgeting with something and was very impulsive. The same symptoms were described in detail, specifically applied to the school environment, by her teacher. These symptoms were also observed in Calliope's interview, with her unable to stay on topic, interrupting the conversation repeatedly, fidgeting constantly and answering impulsively before the questions were finished.

Calliope had witnessed domestic violence at home, up until she had left aged six years old. She was also hit regularly with a stick by her mother's partners. However, in terms of specific trauma symptoms, Calliope denied that she had intrusions in the shape of flashbacks or nightmares related to the abuse. Calliope was not in a constant state of hyperarousal nor did she avoid triggers for her memories, such as visiting the area where she used to live with her mother.

A formulation for Calliope attempted to explain what risk factors predisposed Calliope to present in such a way. Perhaps more salient than the fact that she was in care, was a history of mental health problems in the family, specifically neurodevelopmental problems, which we know have a heritable risk. It is likely that her mother had undiagnosed ADHD, and her siblings had already been identified with the disorder. It is also known that drug taking and alcohol exposure during pregnancy can affect neurodevelopment, and although the specific effects of this are rather unclear (see above) this may have made any pre-existing genetic neurodevelopmental vulnerability more marked. Calliope had presented with hyperactivity, impulsivity and problems with concentration from an early age, always at higher levels than expected for a child of her age. The symptoms were present across environments and settings, and although initially she moved foster carer frequently (i.e., some aspects of this presentation could be a response to these moves) she had now been with the same experienced foster carer for two years and the symptoms remained the same. Based on the fact that they were disabling and also impairing her social functioning and learning at school, she received a diagnosis of ADHD. In terms of her behavioural problems, Calliope had not experienced consistent and effective boundaries from sensitive carers, and had had little chance to learn prosocial strategies. Although Calliope suffered neglect and abuse for years until she was taken into care, she was not suffering from post-traumatic stress disorder (PTSD) currently, although she presented with some confusion about her past and why she had been removed from home (and this could be a target for treatment in its own right, with therapeutic life-story work).

The main precipitant factor (triggering) for her increased behavioural problems (ADHD was present all along and so was a predisposing factor for her current problems) could be that she had just moved to secondary school, where there were more social and academic challenges, and so she was maybe experiencing more frustration because of the challenge keeping up with the lessons. She was also entering adolescence, where hormonal changes and identity issues can prove a combination that affects young people, and especially those who are looked after due to a search for belonging and uncertainty about their life story.

In terms of perpetuating factors (issues that make the problems stay) untreated ADHD can exacerbate a range of social, academic and behavioural issues, for example, ADHD can isolate children from their peers due to annoying or inappropriate behaviours. But if effectively treated the child can maximise their learning and their social abilities, even becoming more popular.

Calliope's current foster carer was committed to her and already very good at helping to manage her disruptive behaviours, as evidenced by the fact they had improved when she first moved in with her, so a combination of medication, psychoeducation and the right support at school, together with continued effective and sensitive caregiving, should guarantee the reduction of these behaviours. So this stable foster placement was a resilience factor for Calliope, along with her own qualities of being a bright girl, with a charming personality.

This formulation covers some of the issues likely to be relevant for Calliope and is by no means complete. It may well change with further assessment, new information and changes in her behaviour or environment or indeed response to treatment. It is a work in progress. But what it does is move the discussion beyond a generalised assumption about issues of neurodevelopmental trauma and attachment to think about how the recent change in environment has precipitated an increase in behavioural problems in the context of a pre-existing neurodevelopmental disorder and opens up a range of specific targets for interventions that can test the hypotheses.

Differential susceptibility Box 3.2

Two brothers, aged six and nine, have been living in an adoptive placement for just over three years. They both experienced physical maltreatment and witnessed significant domestic violence, perpetrated against their birth mother by at least two different partners. The older child was described as being scapegoated in the family and suffered a non-accidental injury from the birth father shortly after his brother's birth. So it seems clear the older child received a much greater 'dose' of maltreatment (duration and severity) during their time in the birth family.

What is puzzling the adoptive family is that the older boy seems to be much better adjusted than his younger brother. Their adoptive parents had expected, and been prepared for, the fact that his long exposure to significant maltreatment would have left him traumatised and that there would be a biological legacy of these experiences in his brain and body. But against the odds he seems relatively well adjusted – he plays football in a team and has a solid group of friends he seems to enjoy hanging out with. He has received lots of therapeutic interventions to help him face his traumas and to develop a closer attachment relationship with his carers but has reported not enjoying the therapy – he would sooner go out and kick a ball – and his parents are disappointed not to have noticed any significant improvement in his 'closeness' to them.

In contrast his younger brother is taking up much more of the parents' time at home and also at school, even taking into account his age. He can be very clingy and becomes easily upset, and this upset gives way to anger towards them and he regularly falls out with a steadily reducing set of friends, which the parents have tried very hard to cultivate. This has been very challenging to his parents who had expected to have to focus on the older boy's needs and they worry they have been diverted from this by the younger child's unexpected level of needs.

Of course, this presentation is well-suited to a differential susceptibility conceptualisation. If the older boy is resilient, then even though he has had such a potentially traumatising start in life, he has coped well nonetheless. Importantly, he may not benefit from further interventions because he may already be at or near his optimal level of functioning, despite all that has happened to him. To keep trying to fix him may risk pathologising his 'normal' and could risk putting him off seeking help later on if he needs it then. In contrast, the younger child requires much more focused attention and perhaps a more specialised and tailored parenting approach. This can be very frustrating for parents (and for teachers if they see a similar pattern in school) who may well feel that they have been good enough carers for him – that their committed and sensitive parenting has been sufficient to help the older boy do okay despite all he suffered, but somehow this seems insufficient to help the younger, less 'damaged' one. But, from a differential susceptibility framework, if the younger one is 'an orchid' then good-enough parenting for him may need to be of a different kind than it would be for most children. It may need to be very focused on his specific needs but, if they can get it right for him, which may not be at all easy to achieve, then the benefits could far outweigh those of his older brother. In other words, there are good scientific reasons why one brother has largely escaped the biological legacy of maltreatment and why the other one, with less evidence of maltreatment, may have more biological, social and psychological needs and so require much more effort to reach his potential.

Note

[1] Readers who are interested in thinking about some of the issues of the overextension of ideas in neuroscience into everyday practice may well wish to look at some of the online resources in blogs and on Twitter in which neuroscientists consider some of the more or less outrageous claims attributed to the new science (Neuroskeptic; The Big Think; Neurobonkers; Neurobollocks).

References

Ackerman, J.P., Riggins, T. and Black, M.M. (2010). A review of the effects of prenatal cocaine exposure among school-aged children. *Pediatrics*, 125, 554–565. doi:10.1542/peds.2009-0637.

Allen, G. (2011). *Early intervention: The next steps*. doi: www.gov.uk/government/uploads/system/uploads/attachment_data/file/284086/early-intervention-next-steps2.pdf, (Accessed 7 June 2016).

Andersen, S.L., Tomada, A., Vincow, E.S., Valente, E., Polcari, A. and Teicher, M.H. (2008). Preliminary evidence for sensitive periods in the effect of childhood sexual abuse on regional brain development. *Journal of Neuropsychiatry and Clinical Neurosciences*, 20, 292–301.

Ariel-Shaw, C.A. and McEachern, J.C. (2001). *Toward a Theory of Neuroplasticity*. Psychology Press.

Barrow, M. and Riley, E.P. (2011). Diagnosis of fetal alcohol syndrome: emphasis on early detection. In P.M. Preece and E.P. Riley (eds), Alcohol, drugs and medication in pregnancy: the long term outcome for the child, pp85–107. *Clinics in Developmental Medicine*, 108. London: MacKeith Press.

Belsky, J. and Pluess, M. (2009). Beyond diathesis stress: Differential susceptibility to environmental influences. *Psychological Bulletin*, 135, 885–908.

Belsky, J. and de Haan, M. (2011). Annual Research Review: Parenting and children's brain development: the end of the beginning. *Journal of Child Psychology and Psychiatry*, 52, 409–28.

Belsky, J., Bakermans-Kranenburg, M.J. and van IJzendoorn, M.H. (2007). For better *and* worse: Differential susceptibility to environmental influences. *Current Directions in Psychological Science*, 16, 300–304.

Boyce, W.T. and Ellis, B.J. (2005). Biological sensitivity to context: I. An evolutionary-developmental theory of the origins and functions of stress reactivity. *Development and Psychopathology*, 17, 271–301.

Butler, G. (1998). Clinical formulation. In A.S. Bellack and M. Hersen (eds), *Comprehensive Clinical Psychology*. Oxford: Pergamon.

D'Onofrio, B.M., Singh, A.L., Iliadou, A., Lambe, M., Hultman, C.M., Neiderhiser, J.M., Långström, N. et al. (2010). A quasi-experimental study of maternal smoking during pregnancy and offspring academic achievement. *Child Development*, 81, 80–100.

Dozier, M., Peloso, E., Lewis, E., Laurenceau, J.P. and Levine, S. (2008). Effects of an attachment-based intervention on the cortisol production of infants and toddlers in foster care. *Development and Psychopathology*, 20, 845–859.

Draganski, B., Gaser, C., Busch, V., Schuierer, G., Bogdahn, U. and May, A. (2004). Changes in grey matter induced by training: Newly honed juggling skills show up as a transient feature on a brain-imaging scan. *Nature*, 427, 311–312.

Edwards, R., Gillies, V. and Horsley, N. (in press). Brain science and early years policy: Hopeful ethos or 'cruel optimism'? *Critical Social Policy*, DOI: 10.1177/0261018315574020.

Fisher, P.A., Stoolmiller, M., Gunnar, M.R. and Burraston, B.O. (2007). Effects of a therapeutic intervention for foster preschoolers on diurnal cortisol activity. *Psychoneuroendocrinology*, 32, 892–905.

Gunnar, M.R., Fisher, P.A. and The Early Experience, Stress, and Prevention Network (2006). Bringing basic research on early experience and stress neurobiology to bear on preventive interventions for neglected and maltreated children. *Development and Psychopathology,* 18, 651–677.

Heckman, J. J. (2008). Schools, Skills and Synapses. *Economic Inquiry*, 46 (3), 289–324.

Howard-Jones, P.A. (2014). Neuroscience and education: myths and messages. *Nature Reviews Neuroscience*, DOI: http://dx.doi.org/10.1038/nrn3817

Kim-Cohen, J., Caspi, A., Taylor, A., Williams, B., Newcombe, R., Craig, I.W. and Moffitt, T. E. (2006). MAOA, maltreatment, and gene-environment interaction predicting children's mental health: New evidence and a meta-analysis. *Molecular Psychiatry*, 11, 903–913.

Kuyken, W., Padesky, C.A. and Dudley, R. (2009). *Collaborative Case Conceptualisation: Working Effectively with Clients in Cognitive-Behavioral Therapy*. New York: Guilford Press.

Mace, C. and Binyon, S. (2005). Teaching psychodynamic formulation to psychiatric trainees Part 1: Basics of formulation. *Advances in Psychiatric Treatment*, 11, 416–423

Macneil, C.A., Hasty, M.K., Conus, P. and Burk, M. (2012). Is diagnosis enough to guide interventions in mental health? Using case formulation in clinical practice. *BMC Medicine*, 10: 111. doi: 10.1186/1741-7015-10-111.

McCrory, E., De Brito, S. and Viding, E. (2010). Research Review: The neurobiology and genetics of maltreatment and adversity. *Journal of Child Psychology and Psychiatry*, 15, 1079–1095.

Obradović, J., Bush, N.R., Stamperdahl, J., Adler, N.E. and Boyce, W.T. (2010). Biological sensitivity to context: The interactive effects of stress reactivity and family adversity on socioemotional behavior and school readiness. *Child Development*, 81, 270–89.

Pickett, K.E. and Wakschlag, L.S. (2011). The short-term and long-term developmental consequences of maternal smoking during pregnancy. In P.M. Preece and E.P. Riley (eds), *Alcohol, drugs and medication in pregnancy: the long term outcome for the child*, pp183–196. Clinics in Developmental Medicine No. 108. London: MacKeith Press.

Pollak, S.D. (2008). Mechanisms linking early experience and the emergence of emotions: Illustrations from the study of maltreated children. *Current Directions in Psychological Science*, 17, 370–375.

Pollak, S.D., Nelson, C., Schlaak, M.F., Roeber, B.J., Wewerka, S.S., Wiik, K.L. et al. (2010). Neurodevelopmental effects of early deprivation in post institutionalized children. *Child Development*, 81, 224–236.

Scheffler, R.M., Brown, T.T., Fulton, B.D., Hinshaw, S.P., Levine, P. and Stone, S. (2009). Positive association between attention-deficit/ hyperactivity disorder medication use and academic achievement during elementary school. *Pediatrics*. 2009. doi: 10.1542/peds.2008-1597.

Shonkoff, J.P. and Bales, S.N. (2011). Science does not speak for itself: Translating child development research for the public and its policymakers. *Child Development*, 82, 17–32.

Singer, L.T. and Minnes, S. (2011). Effects of drugs of abuse on the fetus: Cocaine and opiates including heroin. In P.M. Preece and E.P. Riley (eds), *Alcohol, drugs and medication in pregnancy: the long term outcome for the child*, pp130–152. Clinics in Developmental Medicine No. 108. London: MacKeith Press.

Singer, L.T., Nelson, S., Short, E., Min, M.O. and Kirchner, H.L. (2008). Prenatal cocaine exposure: Drug and environmental effects at 9 years. *Journal of Pediatrics*, 153, 105–111. doi:10.1016/j.jpeds.2008.01.001.

Tunc-Ozcan, E., Sittig, L.J., Harper, K.M., Grafand, E.N. and Redei, E.E. (2014). Hypothesis: Genetic and epigenetic risk factors interact to modulate vulnerability and resilience to FASD. *Frontiers in Genetics*; 5:261. DOI: 10.3389/fgene.2014.00261

van Goozen, S.H.M., Fairchild, G., Snoek, H. and Harold, G.T. (2007). The evidence for a neurobiological model of childhood antisocial behavior. *Psychological Bulletin*, 133, 149–82.

van IJzendoorn, M.H., Bakermans-Kranenburg, M.J. and Ebstein, R.P. (2011). Methylation matters in child development: Toward developmental. Behavioral epigenetics. *Child Development Perspectives*, 5 (4), 305–310. DOI: 10.1111/j.1750-8606.2011.00202.x

Widom, C.S. (2012). *Trauma, Psychopathology, and Violence: Causes, Consequences, or Correlates?* Oxford.

Woollett, K. and Maguire, E.A. (2011). Acquiring 'the Knowledge' of London's layout drives structural brain changes. *Current Biology*, 21, 2109–2114.

Woolgar, M. (2013). The practical implications of the emerging findings in the neurobiology of maltreatment for looked after and adopted children: Recognising the diversity of outcomes. *Adoption and Fostering*, 37, 237–252.

4

EARLY INTERVENTION WITH BABIES AND THEIR PARENTS

Robin Balbernie

Introduction

The idea of providing specialised services that target the relationship between caregiver (usually but not invariably a biological parent) and baby or toddler is one that has become increasingly mainstream over the last decade, and clinical provision in the statutory and voluntary sectors has begun to build up. Such early intervention is proactive rather than waiting for a problem to arise. The prime aim is to prevent maltreatment. It is important to have at hand the rationale behind such provision; and the '1001 Critical Days' campaign and the recent APPG Report 'Building Greater Britons' (2015) has triggered a wide surge of interest (www.1001criticaldays.co.uk) that has the potential to open up a lot of opportunities across the United Kingdom. This chapter gives an overview of the reasons for allocating therapeutic resources during pregnancy and infancy rather than only providing the more established and expensive reactive services that pick up the pieces in the following years. As these are preventative services, where the intervention ideally is on the basis of risk, not symptom or damage, and also because the patient is not an individual but rather the caregiving relationship, it will be argued that such provision does not always belong within statutory services but sometimes might be better seen as an independent multidisciplinary team, preferably based close to the families they will serve within a children's centre. The latter increases accessibility, and goes some way to decrease stigma.

The rationale and setting for early intervention

The first two or three years set a stamp on all that comes after, although there is always room for change, by laying down the unconscious foundations upon which all future growth must be constructed. These experiences become the basis for the human software of relationships, including the future response to threat, recorded in procedural, or implicit (unquestioned, inaccessible to language) memory. Humans are 'designed' to be an adaptable species. 'At birth an infant can develop into an infinity of selves, and its brain is equipped to deal with that uncertainty' (Donald, 2001: 211). The early years can either be positive, as when a child gains the resource of being resilient in adversity so that later stressful events become a challenge rather than a trauma, or negative as when early (s)caregiving leaves a 'basic fault' (Balint, 1968) because of too great a discrepancy between the infant's inherent needs and the quality of parenting that was available. The emotional environment of infancy from the baby's point of view this is the relationships with the parents, will be preserved on both a psychological and neurological level, for good or for ill. The caregiving relationship is also the intervention pathway to hope, as: 'The essence of infant mental health work lies within the parent-child relationship' (Solchany and Barnard, 2001: 46). Relationships are the most important factor in a baby's life, literally vital, and this continues ever after.

Babies are born pre-programmed to seek out, respond and adapt to the caregiving relationship. Attachment theory provides a language to describe the broad-brush patterns. This is a biological given, evolution's answer to the prolonged period of helplessness in childhood and the need to adjust to the infinite possibilities created within a family in interaction with the wider culture. The human genetic package transmits initial flexibility and the capacity to adapt to the environment, fine-tuned by epigenetic processes (Meaney, 2013). Evolutionary success for humans is adaptation to the immediate culture and unforeseeable social diversity rather than to the ecosystem. 'The human brain is the only brain in the biosphere whose potential cannot be realised on its own. It needs to become part of a network before its design features can be expressed' (Donald, 2001: 324). Thus the genetic 'imperative' for the baby is 'fit into what you find', and what a baby is geared to find are relationships.

Babies cannot wait or stand up for themselves. In addition, babies have no comparisons and the quality of caregiving is the major component of their world. Active, satisfying and reciprocal relationships with parents create the 'taken for granted' basis of a sense of identity, self-esteem, appreciation of others, ethical behaviour and self-control. 'Human relationships, and the effects of relationships on relationships, are the building blocks of healthy development. From the moment of conception to the finality of death, intimate and caring relationships are the fundamental mediators of successful human adaptation' (Shonkoff and Phillips, 2000: 27). More than that, the quality and content of the baby's relationship with his or her parents has an effect on the neurobiological structure of the growing child's brain that may be enduring.

Any system is at its most flexible whilst it is being built; and brains under construction automatically adapt to the experiences that follow on from the quality of the caregiving relationship so that 'the infant's transactions with the early socioemotional environment indelibly influence the evolution of brain structures responsible for the individual's socioemotional functioning for the rest of the lifespan' (Schore, 1994: 540). The brain has most neuroplasticity during these first 1001 critical days. Having begun in utero, the post-term period is marked by an immense proliferation and then pruning of synapses, occurring in sequence as different functional capacities wire up. (See Gerhardt, 2015 and Hart, 2006 for good introductions to neurodevelopment.) The genetically governed huge potential number of axons and dendrites (linked by neurotransmitters in the synapses) *must* be slimmed down to be more efficient and to fit the space available, a process that starts with relatively few pre-specifications of detail and ends with neural networks exquisitely adapted to the characteristics of the environment.

Experience-expectant brain growth takes place when the brain is primed to receive particular classes of external information in order to build basic survival skills in the most appropriate way. Neural connections become stabilised and myelinated with use: excited together, united together. The process of pruning is a matter of responding to the environment, whilst its effects depend on the area of the brain in which it occurs. The greatest over-abundance of synapses occurs during sensitive periods, windows of opportunity. The 'fittest', or most used and useful, synapses are selected; and in neural development this is a matter of the level of electrical activity and neurotransmitter production. A matter of 'use it or lose it' is fine in most situations but carries scary implications where there is maltreatment. Pruning in areas involved with higher cognitive functions also occurs throughout adolescence when there is a second phase of enhanced neuroplasticity. Experience-dependant brain changes, though, continue throughout life as new skills and knowledge are learnt and circumstances change.

> Every physical feature of the human nervous system – the brain cells, or neurons, that transmit information; their axons and dendrites that reach great distances to connect with one another; the tiny synapses that are the actual sites of connection; and the supporting cells, or glia, that keep it all going metabolically – responds to life experiences and is continually remodeled to adapt to them. The brain changes when you learn to walk and talk; the brain changes when you store a new memory; the brain changes when you figure out if you're a boy or girl; the brain changes when you fall in love or plunge into depression; the brain changes when you become a parent. (Eliot, 2012: 6)

The caregiving relationship has most impact in the very early years of maximum dependency and the baby's mind will come to fit the family environment; if this is hostile or depriving rather than loving, it makes no difference to the mechanism. 'It is now accepted that early childhood abuse specifically alters limbic system maturation, producing neurobiological alterations that act as a biological substrate for a variety of psychiatric consequences. These include affective instability, inefficient stress tolerance, memory impairment, psychosomatic disorders, and dissociative disturbances' (Schore, 2012: 81). Experience might not affect the inherent process or sequence of brain development, but it does make a difference to the final product and how it will be used. 'These early imprints can be remarkably long lasting because very early stressful life experiences have left emotional systems sensitized or desensitized, with permanent, epigenetically induced high-stress reactivity and excessive primary-process negativistic feeling' (Panksepp and Biven, 2012: 434).

Maltreatment that occurs within the family is particularly pernicious as the brain is 'designed' to adapt its structure in response to the environment of significant relationships. An infant who has developed very insecure attachment has, by the age of one year, encoded what could be lifelong expectations of the world and of the self (this does not mean that later intervention cannot help). In attachment theory the unconscious software of the self is called an internal working model, and this can be locked in self-protective mode. 'Repeated experiences of terror and fear can be engrained within the circuits of the brain as states of mind. With chronic occurrence, these states can become more readily activated (retrieved) in the future, so that they become characteristic traits of the individual' (Siegel, 2012: 55). A survival state has become a personality trait and the capacity to handle any strong emotion in a prosocial manner compromised – and the harmful changes in brain structure and function associated with this are simply 'adaptive responses to an early environment characterised by threat' (McCrory et al., 2010: 1088). The older the child becomes then the harder (and less cost-effective, see http://heckmanequation.org/) it can be to 'rewire' certain areas of the brain, which means that without intervention a child who has experienced abuse or neglect as an infant may unwittingly continue with patterns of responses that are engraved in the mind, even if circumstances change.

The quality of the first relationship with caregivers also affects how a selection of an individual's genes are 'expressed' (switched on or off), setting the limits of what will or will not be possible in the future on a basic biological level. What are called 'epigenetic mechanisms' may alter a gene's function without affecting its sequence (only the sequence is inherited), and these have the capacity to change gene expression in response to environmental pressures, a rapid form of structural adaptation, by adding a chemical signature above the gene that can determine whether or not, or when, it is expressed. Collectively these signatures or markers are known as the epigenome, and its task is to program the genome (Champagne, 2015). Epigenetic markers switch functional characteristic of the gene on and off by controlling how much protein is manufactured. Studies have now shown that 'the epigenome of a prenatally developing infant is sensitive to the mother's experiences, the prenatal environment, and even the experience of birth' (Roth and Sweatt, 2011: 404). Thus experiences of maternal stress, chronic anxiety or restricted diet may have caused epigenetic changes in utero, leading to later negative traits in the child. This is important information for those working with fostering and adoption. Early removal from a high-risk situation does not guarantee a lack of later emotional difficulty, and delay between removal and final placement is also a source of stress (Raine, 2013) that may cause long-lasting epigenetic changes. On the other hand: 'abundant maternal care sets in motion a series of epigenetic changes in gene-expression patterns that make "well-loved" animals more resilient with robust, life-long resistance against various stressors' (Panksepp and Biven, 2012: 308).

Attachment theory has provided a framework for studies on both the immediate and long-term effects of early family experiences on the developing child. Attachment research has integrated the psyche with the outer world of behaviour to demonstrate that 'the patterning or organization of attachment relationships during infancy is associated with characteristic processes of emotional regulation, social relatedness, access to autobiographical memory, and the development of self-reflection and narrative' (Siegel, 1999: 67).

Secure attachment is a protective factor, conferring confidence and adaptability, and without this emotional resource of resilience, neither child nor adult will feel free to make the most of life's possibilities. Secure children and adults can self-repair. An insecure child has too many anxieties that get in the way of investigating the world, so horizons stay reassuringly near. Insecure attachment is a risk factor that will interact with other risks present in the environment of the growing child; the level of attachment disturbance is equivalent to a level of vulnerability that may be difficult to change without help. Children with problems related to insecure attachment begin to soak up statutory resources from early on. Disorganised attachment, frequently a marker for maltreatment, predominates in children referred to CAMHS (Green et al., 2007) and children in special educational provision, many of whom have 'a hard-drive failure that can trip the circuit on violence' (Raine, 2013: 180). The different categories of insecure attachment predispose towards specific difficulties in later life.

Disorganised attachment occurs when the parent either has so many unresolved emotional issues from their own past that there is no mental space left over for their baby or poses some form of threat. In either case the caregiver is unable to soothe, comfort and contain their anxious child and so the attachment system remains in overdrive. Fear has come to be associated with parental behaviour since the attachment system cannot be deactivated in the presence of the putative caregiver. This clash between biology and psychology is not solely a matter of 'obvious' maltreatment, but may occur when 'disrupted parental responses to infant attachment behavior are extreme enough, and contradictory enough, that avoidant or ambivalent strategies cannot be organized in relation to the caregiver; that is, such strategies do not work well enough to maintain a modicum of proximity and protection' (Lyons-Ruth and Jacobvitz, 2008: 675). Such a pattern of interaction can be difficult to recognise and treat as no immediate trauma may be visible; and if it derives from conflictual relationships in the caregiver's own childhood, a 'ghost in the nursery' (Fraiberg, 1980), then infant-parent psychotherapy, perhaps over an extended period of time, may be necessary to address such unconscious dynamics.

The main aim of all forms of early intervention is to prevent or ameliorate the many different parenting conditions that may lead to disorganised attachment. From an evolutionary perspective, the caregiving environment is preparing the child with the skills and traits that will help him or her survive to reproductive age. Any service that reduces the possibility of persisting relationship-based stress during infancy has the potential to reduce the long-term cost to both the individual and society. But at the same time it is important to keep in mind those other, less visible paths to disorganised attachment that will have a similar effect on the developing child's behaviour in the long term.

Child maltreatment does not appear out of the blue, and older children who come into the child protection system almost always have a history of grief going back to babyhood. Early intervention, where vulnerable and over-stressed parents can be identified and supported before the baby suffers and before their own emotionally barren and terrifying past becomes entangled in the relationship (and expectations) with their baby, is an essential preventative measure if we want to avoid a steady growth in the number of referrals to adult mental health services. Taking disorganised attachment as a marker for child abuse (but not assuming flagrant abuse always lies behind it), or its precursors, makes it an important target for preventative services which can then begin at conception.

By recognising that the parent–infant relationship is the crucible for change and development we can look beyond individuals to the wider conditions that impinge upon this relationship. A consideration of reasons removes blame. Every parent always does the best they can for their baby within what is possible for them. A broader perspective, trying to understand rather than passing judgement, points to the importance of known risk factors. It is feasible to anticipate what sort of situation might lead to insecure attachment, and thus offer intervention before anything goes drastically wrong. That is, before responses get so 'hard-wired' into the brain that they become increasingly difficult to change.

There is a large body of research on risk factors, with general agreement on what these are and how they affect parenting (e.g. Fonagy and Higgitt, 2000; Karr-Morse and Wiley, 1997 and 2012; Sameroff, 2000; Zeanah et al., 1997). The Adverse Childhood Experiences Study (www.acestudy.org) shows how a build-up of risks in the family environment is a predictor for, amongst other things, serious physical and mental ill heath, being both a perpetrator and victim of domestic violence and substance abuse (Felitti et al., 1998). These dangers are easily spotted. The parent–baby relationship is always located in a much wider ecological context within which are found both risk and protective factors. These can harm the baby directly but mostly are titrated into the relationship via their effects on the parents' functioning, since they dictate the baby's immediate experiences. The Millennium Cohort Study has confirmed that: 'The greater the number of risks experienced by the child, the greater the problems that the child will face during the lifecourse' (Sabates and Dex, 2012: 22). (For a working list of risks see Appendix 2c of 'Conception to age 2: The age of opportunity' (2013) www.wavetrust.org/our-work/publications).

The research on risk factors means that babies who might have unfortunate developmental pathways through life, because of stresses in their initial relationship with their parents, can often be identified early on. Even the unborn child cannot be assumed to be safe (www.beginbeforebirth.org). The foetus can be directly harmed by a number of toxins (alcohol being a major one as is the effect of stress on the mother) which can cause disability, regulatory disorders, attention difficulties or skill deficits; any one of which may make it hard for the neonate to settle into an attachment relationship. 'Children born already impaired are more likely to be the brunt of destructive parenting behaviours and abuse' (Karr-Morse and Wiley, 1997: 55). A vulnerable baby does not have to experience distress and damage before help is offered. The greater the number of risk factors found in a family's total ecology then the greater the need for immediate assistance. But sadly, the more a family is under stress then the harder it becomes to make full use of any help available. Only a relationship can change a relationship, but if you are ground down by inner and outer circumstances a new relationship is hard to contemplate; and when it is offered it may be harder to trust. Thus, having 'mental health' in the title of any service is a bad start as it carries inevitable stigma.

However, along with pressures on the caregiving relationship there will always be strengths that can be built upon. Improving parenting capability, if it is to be positive for the family, must also build upon the protective factors within and around the caregivers, a task that children's centres excel at. To promote infant well-being, it is necessary to promote the sensitivity and proficiency of both parents. If a family is targeted for services solely on the basis of the risk factors that are known to correlate with child maltreatment, this may indeed employ scarce resources for those most in need, but on the other hand it might alienate families for fear of being labelled potential 'bad' parents or possible abusers. This may be an insoluble dilemma. Risks identify vulnerability; they are not an infallible forecast of disaster. And maltreatment occurs in high-income families with all the advantages of life. This means that interventions must have a strength-based orientation (not solely a deficit model) which has the potential to be more inclusive, with a better capacity to engage with partner agencies in the community using a resilience perspective that can help everyone involved see how their work can contribute to preventing maltreatment. Starting from a protective factor angle, children's centres engaged with the local community are central to prevention, although this cannot be done in the best possible way unless they have a well-qualified multidisciplinary team that preferably includes infant mental health specialists.

Getting the first, prototypical, important relationship of anyone's life more or less right is a necessity, not a luxury. This is the most sensible, kindest and economic time to put in therapeutic resources. Furthermore, unique to this stage of life, one can guarantee that the child both wants to cooperate and has not got stuck in the trap of gaining self-esteem from antisocial acts. This therapeutic window of opportunity is society's best chance to help itself.

Infant mental health teams could be a universal statutory provision set alongside CAMHS, financed by taking two-fifths of any funding allocated to the IAPT for 0–5s initiative (or one-ninth of the total budget), preferably with a well-demarcated cordon sanitaire between them. But if part of a perinatal team, where the work would be limited to mothers (and hopefully fathers) with a serious mental health problem and referrals on the basis of risk are scarce, then this would be best held within adult services. But unless there is uniformity in the structure and management of early intervention teams it might be too risky to leave such an important resource to the vagaries of managers in a large bureaucratic organisation under constant threat of cuts that limit flexibility.

An obvious problem for CAMHS is that in early intervention, which can begin during pregnancy and continue up until at least the second birthday, there is no individually identified patient. The 'patient' is the caregiving relationship, which hopefully includes both mother and father and all that their backgrounds and the individual baby together contribute. But parents must choose to be engaged. Also, any file needs to be opened in their name not the child's, both for clear ethical reasons and for any child protection concerns (there may be children with different surnames in the same family, or children waiting to be born) as well as ease of communication with adult services when they are involved – as is normal practice in children's centres. Keeping files in the baby's name has one advantage though. Since they do not say much, notes will be sparse, as otherwise confidential third party information from the parents is being recorded where the child will one day have a right of access. Plus, who in their right mind would knowingly want any baby to collect a mental health record? This then deprives any CAMHS of numbers, so may be resisted by managers as not contributing to targets they are forced to meet.

Infant mental health intervention is a highly skilled speciality but many professions are involved. The number of qualified practitioners in infant–parent psychotherapy is steadily growing with courses available through the Anna Freud Centre, OXPIP, the Tavistock Centre and the School of Infant Mental Health. These are post-professional qualification trainings, psychodynamically based, and a properly trained clinician merits a high pay band, anathema in the current climate of frugality where CAMHS managers are reducing the grade and pay of the most qualified and experienced clinicians wherever they can. But you do not have to be a psychotherapist to be an infant mental health specialist; and there are other equally useful interventions such as Interaction Guidance and therapeutic groups along the lines of Mellow Parenting and Circle of Security. Midwives and health visitors (the best early warning system for adult problems) are central as they are universal, and both are specialising in early detection and intervention with vulnerable families. An infant mental health team has to be multidisciplinary and a relationship-based organisation (Bertacci, 1996), again quite contrary to the frantic pressure of a reduced CAMHS faced with more referrals than they can hope to offer an adequate service to; and in the same spirit, treatment must follow the caregiving relationships rather than a formula and so, in some cases, might need to be open-ended; such a cavalier attitude to the ethos of meeting targets may cause organisational stress and bad feeling.

There is a tendency for CAMHS services to be largely clinic-based. They generally do less home visiting than adult teams or community workers from a children's centre. This is hardly the best place to work with a vulnerable family where the normal heightened stress and anxiety caused by a new baby is amplified by the sense of being judged, let alone the anxieties that can arise in a noisy waiting room; and CAMHS might have negative associations for the parent. Better for the clinician to contain the anxiety of a home visit (unless unsafe), where more can be learned from a single observation than a string of clinic sessions, than the parents having the hassle of transporting an infant, plus all the attendant clobber and possibly a sibling. Another reason to keep infant mental health services distant from CAMHS is that almost invariably the family has not requested help, it has been suggested by some professional such as a midwife, health visitor or children's centre worker. Every referral to CAMHS has motivated parents asking for their child to be 'fixed'; in infant mental health there is usually no child with a symptom (though babies can have many emotional difficulties, primarily reactive) as the prime aim is to maintain healthy social and emotional development as far as possible. At this age most 'problems' begin as an intangible within the caregiving relationships that, as a risk analysis shows, can have a multitude of sources. This is why an early intervention team needs to both be highly skilled, close, creative and multidisciplinary; and the nature of the personal commitment to this work, with more stress and less waiting times, demands an organisationally unruly team – if not there is a problem. In some regions, depending on managerial reflectiveness and attachment category, such a team may be more efficient and creative in the voluntary sector (see www.pipuk.org.uk) and feel more supported and contained within the focused and skilled bustle of a children's centre.

There is a breadth of evidence-based practice in the field of early intervention; although, based on the 'gold standard' of RCTs, some of the population level effects are small (For examples see www.aimh.org.uk). One reason for this is that poverty, which amplifies and concentrates all the other risks, remains the source of major stress on parents and all the psychological interventions in the world will not affect that. This diversity shows the necessity for setting up appropriately trained teams housing multiple skills rather than sticking to a single method of offering 'therapeutic' help to vulnerable families. An important caveat is that virtually all the intervention research has been done with mothers, with the reality of the significance of fathers somewhat side-lined; but see Zero to Three, May 2015, (35) 5 as a corrective.

Well-planned, well-funded services with practice-based evidence to back them up can redirect a likely developmental pathway along a new, healthier direction. 'Programs that combine child-focussed educational activities with explicit attention to parent-child interaction patterns and relationship building appear to have the greatest impacts' (Shonkoff and Phillips, 2000: 379). Whereas 'services that are supported by more modest budgets and are based on generic support, often without a clear delineation of intervention strategies matched directly to measurable objectives, appear to be less effective for families facing significant risk' (ibid). Babies cannot wait and they need the best, and stressed parents need time. It takes time to build the relationship that is needed to change a relationship, and if your background has given you an association between close and 'caring' relationships and maltreatment then interest and kindness can be frightening – 'We cannot interrupt cycles of disorganised attachment unless we provide a haven of safety for mothers' (Slade and Sadler, 2013: 34). Treatment during this period can be rather artificially divided between individual and group as well as home or centre based, a necessary flexibility.

One way of approaching all forms of early intervention is through the lens provided by the concept of 'reflective function', a parental capacity that promotes and fuses with secure attachment. 'Secure attachment and reflective function are overlapping constructs, and the vulnerability associated with insecure attachment lies primarily in the child's diffidence in conceiving of the world in terms of psychic rather than physical reality' (Fonagy et al., 2002: 351). To a large extent the parents' capacity for reflecting on their own relationships and the fact that mental states lie behind all behaviour is a signifier for the level of security of attachment that their children have with them. Both infant parent psychotherapy and all the diverse brands of video feedback (e.g. McDonough, 2004; Juffer et al., 2007) are different ports of entry into the parents' internal representations of their infant, providing the opportunity to free up and improve the observational skills, empathy and appropriate responsiveness that are usually so taken for granted as to go unnoticed. 'A caretaker with a predisposition to see relationships in terms of mental content permits the normal growth of the infant's mental function. His or her mental state anticipated and acted on, the infant will be secure in attachment' (Fonagy et al. 1991: 214). In other words, a positive intersubjective overlap, or 'limbic resonance' (Lewis et al., 2000), leads to healthy emotional development. An improvement in reflective function may lie behind all successful interventions that aim to improve the sensitive and appropriate responsiveness that is one basis of secure attachment.

An infant mental health team needs to call upon a wide range of skills and strategies that together 'contribute to the parent's understanding of the infant, the awakening or repair of the early developing attachment relationship, and the parent's capacity to nurture and protect a young child' (Weatherston, 2000: 6). This means strengthening all relationships, whether between parent and child, therapist and parents or within the boundaries of the service. Starting from the fundamental premise that all parents want to do the best they can for their babies but differ in their access to internal and external resources, an early intervention team builds on strengths in order to remove any obstacles that get in the way of everyday parenting. A parenting class is often inappropriate as parents, unsurprisingly, may not appreciate the assumption that they just need 'training'; indeed, such an attitude: 'may send a message of presumed incompetence, which might undermine a mother's or father's self-confidence and contribute inadvertently to less effective performance' (Shonkoff and Phillips, 2000: 371). Infant mental health specialists need to be experts – but they should always relate to parents on the basis of partnership and strengths, not authority and failure, modelling the relationships they wish to promote.

References

Balint, M. (1968). *The Basic Fault*. London: Tavistock Publications.

Bertacci, J. (1996). Relationship-based organizations. *Zero to Three*, 17 (2), 1–7.

Champagne, F.A. (2015). Epigenetics of the developing brain. *Zero to Three*, 35 (3), 2–8.

Donald, M. (2001). *A Mind So Rare*. New York: W.W. Norton and Co.

Eliot, L. (2012). *Pink Brain Blue Brain*. Oxford: Oneworld.

Felitti, V.S., Anda, R.F., Nordenburg, D., Williamson, D.F., Spitz, A.M., Edwards, V., Koss M.P. and Marks, J.S. (1998). Relationship of childhood abuse and household dysfunction to many of the leading causes of death in adults. *American Journal of Preventive Medicine*, 14 (4), 245–247.

Fonagy, P., Gergely, G., Jurist, E.L. and Target, M. (2002). *Affect Regulation, Mentalization, and the Development of the Self*. New York: Other Press.

Fonagy, P. and Higgitt, A. (2000). An attachment theory perspective on early influences on development and social inequalities in health. pp. 521–578 in: Osofsky, J.D. and Fitzgerald, H.E. (eds) *WAIMH Handbook of Infant Mental Health*, Vol. 4: Infant Mental Health in Groups at High Risk. New York: John Wiley and Sons.

Fonagy, P., Steele, H., Steele, M., Moran, G.S. and Higgitt, A.C. (1991). The capacity for understanding mental states: The reflective self in parent and child and its significance for security of attachment. *Infant Mental Health Journal*, 12 (3), 201–218.

Fraiberg, S. (ed.) (1980) *Clinical Studies in Infant Mental Health*. New York: Basic Books.

Gerhardt, S. (2015). *Why Love Matters*. London: Routledge.

Green, J., Stanley, C. and Peters, S. (2007). Disorganized attachment representations and atypical parenting in young school age children with externalising disorder. *Attachment and Human Development*, 9 (3), 207–222.

Hart, S. (2006). *Brain, Attachment, and Personality*. London: Karnac.

Karr-Morse, R. and Wiley, M.S. (1997). *Ghosts From the Nursery: Tracing the Roots of Violence*. New York: The Atlantic Monthly Press.

Karr-Morse, R. and Wiley, M.S. (2012). *Scared Sick: The Role of Childhood Trauma in Adult Disease*. New York: Basic Books.

Lewis, T., Amini, F. and Lannon, R. (2000). *A General Theory of Love*. New York: Vintage Books.

Lyons-Ruth, K. and Jacobvitz, D. (2008). Attachment disorganization: Genetic factors, parenting contexts, and developmental transformation from infancy to adulthood. pp. 666–697 in: Cassidy, J. and Shaver, P.R. (eds) *Handbook of Attachment: Theory, Research, and Clinical Applications*. 2nd. New York: The Guilford Press.

McDonough, S. (2004). Interaction guidance: promoting and nurturing the caregiving relationship. pp. 79–96 in: Sameroff, A.J., McDonough, S.C. and Rosenblum, K.L. (eds) *Treating Parent–Infant Relationship Problems: Strategies for Intervention*. New York: The Guilford Press.

McCrory, E.J., De Brito, S. and Viding, E. (2010). Research review: The neurobiology and genetics of maltreatment and adversity. *The Journal of Child Psychology and Psychiatry,* 51(10), 1079–1095.

Meaney, M.J. (2013). *Epigenetics and the Environmental Regulation of the Genome and its Function.* pp. 99–128 in: Narvaez, D., Panksepp, J., Schore, A. N. and Gleason, T. R. (eds) *Evolution, Early Experience and Human Development.* Oxford: Oxford University Press.

Panksepp, J. and Biven, L. (2012). *The Archaeology of Mind: Neuroevolutionary Origins of Human Emotions.* New York: W.W. Norton and Co.

Raine, A. (2013). *The Anatomy of Violence: The Biological Roots of Crime.* London: Allen Lane, Penguin.

Roth, T.L. and Sweatt, J.D. (2011). Annual Research review: Epigenetic mechanisms and environmental shaping of the brain during sensitive periods of development. *The Journal of Child Psychology and Psychiatry,* 52(4), 398–408.

Sabates, R. and Dex, S. (2012). *Multiple risk factors in young children's development.* CLS Cohort Studies. Working paper 2012/1. Downloaded from www.cls.ioe.ac.uk/

Sameroff, A. (2000) *Ecological perspectives on developmental risk.* pp. 1–33 in: Osofsky, J.D. and Fitzgerald, H.E. (eds) *WAIMH Handbook of Infant Mental Health,* Vol. 4: Infant Mental Health in Groups at High Risk. New York: John Wiley and Sons.

Schore, A.N. (1994) *Affect Regulation and the Origin of the Self: The Neurobiology of Emotional Development.* New Jersey: Erlbaum.

Schore, A. (2012) *The Science of the Art of Psychotherapy.* New York: W.W. Norton and Co.

Siegel, D.J. (1999) *The Developing Mind: Towards a Neurobiology of Interpersonal Experience.* New York: The Guilford Press.

Siegel, D.J. (2012) *The Developing Mind.* New York: The Guilford Press.

Shonkoff, J. P. and Phillips, D.A. (eds) (2000) *From Neurons to Neighbourhoods: The Science of Early Childhood Development.* National Research Council and Institute of Medicine Committee on Integrating the Science of Early Childhood Development. Board on Children, Youth and Families, Commission on Behavioral and Social Sciences and Education. Washington D. C.: National Academy Press.

Slade, A. and Sadler, L. (2013) Minding the baby: Complex trauma and home visiting. *International Journal of Birth and Parent Education,* 1(1), 32–35.

Solchany, J.E. and Barnard, K.E. (2001) Is mom's mind on her baby? Infant mental health in Early Head Start. *Zero to Three,* 22(1), 39–47.

Weatherston, D.J. (2000) The infant mental health specialist. *Zero to Three,* 21(2), 3–10.

Zeanah, C.H., Boris, N.W. and Larrieu, J.A. (1997) Infant development and developmental risk: A review of the past ten years. *Journal of the American Academy of Child and Adolescent Psychiatry,* 32, 165–178.

5

THE VIEW FROM THE BRIDGE: BRINGING A THIRD POSITION TO CHILD HEALTH

Sebastian Kraemer

Introduction

A mental health presence in hospital paediatrics adds an extra player to the medical partnership with patients and families. Now there are two contrasting kinds of opinion about children and their health disorders, and they are not always compatible. The tension created may cause divisions between staff, but it can also lead to a more three-dimensional view of the patient's predicament.

The ability to take part in triangular relationships is an emotional and intellectual achievement for the developing mind. As the psychoanalyst Ronald Britton put it 'a third position comes into existence [that] provides us with a capacity for seeing ourselves in interaction with others and for entertaining another point of view while retaining our own' (Britton, 1989, p. 87).[1] Likewise it is an enrichment of child health practice when necessary differences between paediatrics and child mental health add depth and perspective to the clinical picture.

A clinical example

Alex is 11 and has asthma. He keeps getting admitted to the paediatric hospital ward from the emergency department (A&E) with dangerous attacks of wheezing. This had happened ten times during the year preceding his referral to me, the trigger for which was a concern about his mother's attitude to his illness. She is obsessed with it, keeping detailed notes of every wheeze.

Together with the referring paediatrician I meet the two of them. Mother explains that doctors in A&E always ask *her* about Alex's symptoms when they should be asking *him*. The trouble is that he would usually say that he was ok even when he was really ill. It's clear that there is a breakdown of trust between mother and the paediatric team.

In the first consultation she is rather prickly and self-righteous both with me and with the paediatrician, but becomes more interested as she follows a conversation between us that reveals our different clinical perspectives. I ask her about Alex growing up and she says 'please not!', which opens up another aspect of their relationship, not about asthma. He is leaving childhood and she does not like it. I suggest they are an 'asthma couple', enmeshed by his illness and her anxiety about it. This uncritical observation seems to make sense to both of them. We hear that Alex's father does not live with him but visits and stays at weekends.

I offer to meet him with them (from then on without the paediatrician) a few weeks later. Father is a big man and looks unusual. It turns out that he is part descended from central Asian people, which explains Alex's appearance – his dark straight hair – which we talk about with enthusiasm. I get the impression that none of this has been discussed in the family, and we enjoy doing so now. Father had never attended an outpatient appointment with his son before, so this consultation brings a third perspective for Alex, now seeing himself in interaction with each parent, and them with each other. Mother is clearly the primary parent, while father is not expected to do much extra. But he is keen to get involved. His entrance at this point in Alex's life is crucial for his development as a soon-to-be adolescent. Once mother's anxiety about the prospect of Alex growing up has been acknowledged the atmosphere in these consultations becomes warm and humorous, and her thoughtful intelligence shines through.

We meet for several further reviews (father only attending once more) at widely spaced intervals during the next 18 months by which time mother has thrown away her notebook. Having already tailed off soon after the first two meetings, Alex's emergency admissions had stopped altogether.

While the reason for this referral was wheezing, its timing[2] was partly determined by Alex's impending adolescence; an alarming

prospect for mother and son. Even if neither of them was thinking about it, both were anxious about what comes next. Here is
one triangle repeated on the vertex of another. Paediatrician and
psychiatrist see the problem differently, as we are bound by training and temperament to do.[3] As mother and son witnessed us working together it became easier for them to take their own positions
alongside ours. When father joined us, more room for change was
opened up within the family.

Since most of the anxiety had been carried by his mother, it
would have been much less productive for me to see Alex on his
own. This kind of intervention is essentially a part of paediatric
practice and not a separate mental health treatment.

Location of the problem: Where is it really?

A serious difficulty in making the case for mental health teams in
paediatrics is that many patients with complex medical presentations do not appear to have mental problems. Rather than being 'all
in the mind' it's all in the body. Even when very ill, Alex was always
cheerful. The predicaments that lead paediatricians to seek our support are often confusing.

If, unlike Alex, a young person presents with mysterious physical symptoms with *no* pre-existing paediatric diagnosis there is an
urgent need to find one. A 14-year-old girl is referred by her GP
to a consultant paediatrician because of dizzy spells and intermit-
tent hearing loss. The paediatrician does her assessment, including
a variety of tests, and finds no abnormality. During the next few
weeks she gets neurological and ENT (ear, nose and throat) opin-
ions, both of which confirm her findings. The neurologist also adds
that in his view this is a psychological problem, which she is beginning to think too. What is the paediatrician to say?

Imagine you are this patient with your mother in the clinic. The
doctor has a hunch that is supported by a more specialist medical
colleague, but it takes her out of her comfortable expertise. She
begins, 'we have done all the tests but found no explanation for
these symptoms'. You hear this and think 'What's wrong with me
then?' As medical uncertainty increases so does the anxiety in the
room. She goes on: 'I think this could be due to some stress or worry
that you are having...' Your silent rumination continues: 'she thinks
that this is all in my mind, that I'm just making it up! (The only

stress I have is from my giddiness)'. Your and your mother's faith in this doctor is shaken; she has failed to find a proper cause, and is now telling you the symptoms are not real.

Although there will be a number of parents or children who are greatly relieved to hear it, the suggestion of a psychological origin for so far unexplained symptoms often creates offence and the risk of humiliation; it both exposes what appear to be the doctor's limitations, and implies that there is something wrong with the child's family. 'The temptation for professionals, unable to diagnose a physical cause, is to blame the child and/or the family as the cause of the problem' (Carter, 2002, p. 38). 'Medically unexplained symptoms' (MUS) has become a category in its own right as if it defined a problem in the patient, like psychosomatic disorder. Though more inclusive than somatisation the term fails to neutralise the stigma of non-medical causes.'[4] This is despite the unconscious irony embedded in the phrase, which clearly does not refer to anything in the patient at all. What MUS describes is a problem in the doctor's mind, not the patient's. By her awkward manner she transfers her frustration – tinged perhaps with shame at not seeming to be a clever enough paediatrician – to the mother, who then feels that she is not a good enough parent. 'Even the most caring physician can be perceived as guilty of an empathic failure when the patient and family believe they are being told that "nothing is wrong" after weeks or months of symptomatic distress and several hours in a waiting room' (Campo and Fritz, 2001, p. 469).[5]

The implications of ascribing a mental origin for a physical symptom introduce an entirely new dimension to the clinical picture.

Body and mind

'Physical disorders are seen as "real" and patients are seen as victims, whereas psychiatric disorders are seen as "not real," and patients are seen as partly responsible for their problems' (Hatcher and Arroll, 2008, p. 1124).

Where does this idea come from? Of course not all referrals face such resistance but the peculiar experience of taking the step from physical to mental is familiar to all of us. It opens up an enormous, disconcerting field to explore. Since at least the European enlightenment[6] the body has been perceived as material; a living thing, but subject to deterministic cause and effect. The mind, on the other hand, is where thoughts, wishes, beliefs, desires, anxieties and dreams are located along, most crucially, with choice. This distinction is most often associated with the philosophy of René Descartes. 'The Cartesian doctrine of the immaterial unextended soul served to open up a space for human freedom which would have been precluded ... if the soul were material' (Wright and Potter, 2000, p. 4).

Descartes' intention was to allow mental events to be detached from physical ones; to show that mind exists without body and to remove any hint of mentality from physical objects (Skirry, 2005). He set out to be more scientific about matter, for example not to ascribe the falling of a stone to its desire to reach the centre of the earth. The body is material, like a machine, but the mind is moral. Many philosophers before Descartes, such as Plato and St Augustine, struggled with various possible relationships between the two, but what they shared is a concept of mind, however connected to it, as a separate entity from the body (Wright and Potter, 2002). This is still the case. We know a lot more about the brain now, including how mental content, such as belief, can have an effect in the body. Good examples are the placebo effect (Mayberg et al., 2002)[7] which, like psychotherapy, alters the brain (Abbas et al., 2014). We always knew that sexual fantasy has bodily effects, and science has caught up with ancient knowledge that you can die from a broken heart (Tennant and McLean, 2001). The interdependence of each domain is no longer challenged. Besides the effects of toxins or drugs on consciousness there are interesting correlations (while not the same as causes) between somatisation disorders and changes in the brain (Spence, 2006). Yet despite scientific advances we stubbornly hold on to a largely unquestioned assumption of the separateness of mind and body, comparable to that between the sexes. As with male–female so with mind–body; you are either in one or in the other. The impact of this tradition on clinical thinking is that we are inclined to see a medical condition as a fault in the machine, while a mental disorder is subject to free will, entailing choice.

To add to the size of the moral landscape revealed, in paediatric practice the problem is now not only seen to be in the child's mind. Responsibility for it extends into the family and beyond. From the point of view of the players in our clinical scenario this is a massive step to take. In a study of paediatric staff's experience with patients who have medically unexplained symptoms Furness et al. conclude, 'Making the transition from physical to psychological care was perceived as one of the most difficult stages in the professional–carer relationship because of parental resistance to giving up the notion of an identifiable, treatable physical cause for the symptoms in favour of an approach addressing psychological and social issues' (Furness et al., 2009, p. 579).

The stigma of mental illness is usually ascribed to prejudice about madness as a dangerous affliction. But in paediatric liaison the principal anxiety is the sudden prospect of having to consider someone's responsibility, even blame, for physical symptoms where none existed before. Doctors tend to think that emotional disorders are not real illnesses because there is no lesion (afflicted tissue) to explain them. Actually mental health practitioners think the same, but usually have better skills in working out where the affliction is to be found, outside the body. *The reality is somewhere else*: often – though not evident in Alex's case – contained in a narrative of intergenerational sorrow, grievance or loss.[8] The fact that neuroscience and immunology can show altered tissues in mental disorders (White et al., 2012; Davison, 2012) might ease the transition, but it does not fully explain them. The binary disjunction between dimensions remains. Psychological therapies only exaggerate it; if there is a mental way out of the problem does that not suggest there was a mental – even wilful – way in?

The development of health professions in modern times has faithfully reflected prevailing notions of mind and body. Whatever integration and 'parity of esteem' we may wish to see between them, the difference between a paediatrician and a psychiatrist is only too real. It would take a cultural revolution of the kind envisaged by Iain McGilchrist in his magisterial text, *The Master and His Emissary: The Divided Brain and the Making of the Western World* (2009), to make the barrier more permeable.

Creating a third position: The true meaning of MUS

The history of the relationship between paediatrics and child psychiatry shows conflict between them from quite early on. In 1931, the Chicago paediatrician Joseph Brenneman wrote 'there is a menace in psychologizing the school child, psychiatrizing his behavior and overorganizing his habits and his play' (Brenneman, 1931, p. 391). A similar antipathy was also evident in British child health. The great paediatrician Sir James Spence (1892–1954)[9] was firmly against the development of child psychiatry as a profession in its own right. In a biographical review written 20 years after his death, Donald Court (also a distinguished paediatrician) wrote '...his intuitive understanding of people made him unwilling to recognize the extent and complexity of mental ill health in children and resistant to the development of child psychiatry as an independent discipline' (Court, 1975, p. 88). Though Spence had been a pioneer in providing room on the wards for mothers to live in with their sick babies, and was clearly sympathetic to the loneliness of child patients in long-stay hospitals (Spence, 1947), he was quite dismissive of the efforts of John Bowlby and James Robertson to show that children in hospital were significantly affected by separation from their parents. In 1951 Robertson was invited to present his observations to the British Paediatric Association. As soon as he had finished Spence was on his feet, asking 'what is wrong with emotional upset?' (Brandon et al., 2009). Robertson records his discouraging discovery that 'the myth of the Happy Children's Ward that has sustained the hospital professions for several decades was very resistant to what I had to say' (Robertson and Robertson, 1989, p. 19). With Bowlby's support, he decided to make a scientific film. When *A Two-Year-Old Goes to Hospital* (1952) was shown at the Royal Society of Medicine in November 1952 'in the discussion which followed, the first reaction of the audience seemed to be a frank refusal to admit that the child was distressed' (Lancet, 1952). Spence was clearly not alone. The paediatric establishment, including children's nurses, was affronted. Three years later, shortly after the first showing of Robertson's film in Scotland, the child psychiatrist Fred Stone was offered a research grant by his colleagues at Glasgow's Royal Hospital for Sick Children to 'disprove all this Bowlby nonsense' (Karen, 1994, pp 80, 81).[10]

Yet there were pioneering efforts in the United States and in Europe to get paediatricians and psychiatrists working together. The child psychiatrist Leo Kanner (1894–1981)[11] writes in strikingly familiar terms about impediments to these ventures. In 1930 a planned 'psychiatric workshop' for paediatric trainees and staff in a clinic at Johns Hopkins hospital 'did not work out too well' (Kanner et al., 1953, p. 394) largely because the doctors were too busy with acute medicine to find the time. He takes an even-handed view of the cultural gap keeping medical and mental apart:

The community child guidance clinics have made great contributions to the understanding of children's feelings and parental attitudes. They were set up as 'teams' of psychiatrist, psychologist and social worker. Pediatricians were left out of the arrangement. ... Insult was added to injury when pediatricians, kept at a distance from all that went on in the clinics, were blamed for their alleged lack of comprehension and interest. Only recently, after about 30 years, have the child guidance clinics begun to show a desire to break through the walls of their isolation from medicine ... Obviously, pediatricians could expect nothing from the pontifical attitude of the community child guidance clinics. (Kanner et al., 1953, p. 394)

Other attempts to introduce mental health skills and knowledge to paediatricians also petered out. There were a variety of reasons for this failure, largely due to the far greater time and emotional pressures on doctors trying to treat behavioural and emotional disorders, but also to 'such puzzlements as how to help parents accept the suggestion that a child be seen by a psychiatrist' (Kanner et al., 1953, p. 396). This remains a problem: '... referrals to psychologists and psychiatrists were perceived by parents as labelling their child as 'mad' or as 'obviously making it up' (OT; Nurse), and could permanently damage the relationship between practitioner and family' (Furness et al., 2009, p. 580).[12] Hinton and Kirk (2016) note that 'referrals to child and adolescent mental health services are often a last resort when other approaches have failed'.

My colleague who was looking after Alex, the asthmatic boy presented above, told me afterwards that she had only been able to refer him to me once she had become quite exasperated by his mother. Her wish to keep on cordial terms with the family was trumped by a fear that her patient could die. Despite her good working relationship with me, resistance to crossing the body–mind boundary was great. Without our collegial friendship the referral might well not have taken place at all. In view of the evident strengths in the family and their exceptional responsiveness to therapeutic consultations, that could have been tragic.

In many parts of the world, there are now thriving partnerships between paediatricians and mental health specialists (Pinsky et al., 2015;[13] Edwards and Titman, 2010), some well established in centres of excellence, but they are in a minority (Slowick and Noronha, 2004; Woodgate and Garralda, 2006).[14] Liaison teams in general hospitals are less secure, easily broken up when committed enthusiasts move on. In Britain there are special interest groups of mental health professionals working in paediatrics but their collective voice is weak in a National Health Service driven by contracts and outcomes (and intimidated by shrinking budgets) rather than by service and patient needs. The trend towards highly regulated training and evidence-based practice has kept us apart in our different professional bodies; paediatrics, psychiatry, psychology, child mental health, nursing, individual and family psychotherapies in particular. In none of these disciplines is paediatric mental health a mandatory element in training. Just as in the United States 80 years ago community child and adolescent mental health clinics in Britain now are relatively exclusive (and overworked) organisations with preoccupations far from hospitals and child health. Meanwhile (with honourable exceptions), the paediatric establishment has largely dedicated itself to what most people expect it to do, which is to focus on the diagnosis and treatment of physical disease.[15] Despite many official working parties and recommendations over the years,[16] there is little sign of a national understanding of this complex story: 'Repeated exhortations for cross-agency collaboration are faithfully incorporated into national guidance and protocols but have not had much impact on commissioning. Institutional resistance does not disappear because documents say it should... It is as if child mental health practice had opened a previously unknown room in the paediatric house to reveal quite new kinds of anxiety and sorrow in the complex lives of children' (Kraemer, 2009, p. 571).

An 'institutional blind spot' remains (Kraemer, 2015). A critical mass for creating joined up working has not yet been achieved, leaving the child health professions in a collective state of ambivalence. In too many places paediatricians have been disappointed by the lack of readily accessible mental health colleagues to work with. They have had to manage on their own or beg for help from hard-pressed local CAMHS. Given high thresholds for access to these services, children referred to them with puzzling medical symptoms may be given a low priority – with a long wait and little chance of a joint consultation – or not be accepted at all, as happens to many children referred.[17]

Without first-hand experience of an effective partnership – likened to a marriage[18] – paediatricians are in no position to spell out to colleagues, managers and commissioners what they need.

Neither frustration nor ignorance is a sufficient basis for designing new services. Kanner's prescient observation from the 1950s about the paediatrician in need of a mental health opinion for a patient is still valid:

> There is a choice between 3 possibilities: one is that these needs are disregarded or handled clumsily to the patients' detriment. Another possibility is that these children are sent away to be treated elsewhere;[19] this deprives the pediatricians of valuable experience. A third alternative presents itself in the form of a psychiatric unit in the children's hospital. (Kanner et al., 1953, p. 397)

To return to our harassed paediatrician with the deaf and dizzy patient; clearly the best choice is Kanner's 'third alternative'. Once she has explored the medical options she can then discuss the patient with the mental health team to work out a strategy for referral. In a case of this kind, letters or emails tend to screen out the most revealing and useful information; a conversation is required. This can be in the corridor (as happened in this case), in a visit to the mental health team's own meeting, or in the weekly multidisciplinary meeting of all staff where there is space to reflect on complex cases. It is easier to say than to write 'I was pretty sure this is psychological; there was something about the way the mother and child interacted which made me feel uneasy, as if mother was somehow encouraging her daughter's problem.' The paediatrician decided that she would say to the girl and her mother: 'I am puzzled about these symptoms. We have done enough tests for now, so I am going to need some help to look at this a different way. I have been talking to my colleague X who is a specialist in this kind of problem. I want him to join me to help me work out what's needed here'. The moment of truth is the mention of X's profession which may include the terms 'mental' or 'psycho-' in it.[20] Some families will bristle even at this diplomatic proposal but it helps that the doctor, while introducing a third point of view, is taking a one-down position. She makes herself part of the problem; the true meaning of MUS. At the same time she demonstrates that she knows and trusts this new kind of specialist and will not abandon the family to yet another consultation where they have to tell the story all over again. Speaking in 2010 at the launch of his report on the needs of children in the NHS Sir Ian Kennedy said, 'No 21st century health system should require parents and children to go from place to place or even worse to go to multiple appointments to tell the same story' (Kennedy, 2010).

If it is to have a chance of success the vital feature of this step is that it is not done in parallel with any other search for help. Asking for a further expert opinion at the same time clouds the moment. If not distracted by yet more medical tests the view from the fragile bridge between body and mind can open the minds of all players to something new and provisional. 'The development of a third position ... is a necessary preliminary to the sceptical position' (Britton, 2015, p. 81).

Conclusion: Liaison is an end in itself

There is no doubting the need for a mental health presence in paediatrics. Epidemiological studies show that children with chronic disease and/or medically unexplained symptoms have higher rates of mental disorder than the general population (Meltzer et al., 2000;[21] Hysing et al., 2007;[22] Garralda and Rask, 2015).[23] There is a large literature of psychological interventions for children of all ages with unexplained symptoms, with and without underlying physical illness.[24] Neither neuroscience nor philosophy play much part in this knowledge, most of which depends on a developmental view of children's and parents' experiences of illness, anxiety, pain and disability. A clue to the origins of somatisation (Rask et al., 2013) may better found in the normal state of a human infant who has never heard of Descartes, one whose mind and body have not yet been partitioned.

Once a mental health colleague is engaged it is often possible (as in Alex's case) for the patient and family to continue consultations without the paediatrician, but she still carries overall responsibility for the patient's care. She remains in the mind of the mental health clinician who is all the while providing a service *both to the family and to the paediatric department*. This triangular set up is a necessary condition for good liaison. Modern health services have difficulty promoting partnerships of this kind, preferring 'patient pathways' which risk prejudging the intervention required (and a premature entrance through the wrong door) rather then reflecting on it. Disintegration of comprehensive services for the sake of contracting does not do justice to the actual experience of a child and family in confused clinical situations.

A passing opportunity to enlist a mental health point of view is easily lost by thoughtless adherence to protocols.

Though it is essential to collect clinical activity data, the quality of the resulting service cannot be judged by measurable outcomes alone. The liaison relationship is an end in itself. Having evolved in the context of multiple caregiving (Hrdy, 2016) all humans are programmed to monitor relationships between significant others. Our survival as small children depends on trusting partnerships amongst caregivers. Supporting Britton's formulation in the laboratory, Fivaz-Depeursinge et al. (2012) show how acutely attentive infants are to the way their parents are getting on. Likewise, patients and families are attuned to the quality of professional discourse in a paediatric department, for example the extent to which clinical staff can entertain multiple explanations for child health problems. This capacity is fostered in regular multidisciplinary meetings where colleagues are free to speak their minds (Kraemer, 2010) to get a sense of a child's experience of illness from all sides. Another voice resonating from the past is that of Sir Harry Platt (1886–1986), the orthopaedic surgeon who chaired the report on the welfare of children in hospital usually named after him: 'What, after all, is it really like to be that child in this hospital, at this moment?" (Platt, 1959).

As it did for Alex, the inclusion of mental health in paediatric practice can reduce hospital admissions and unnecessary investigations. It may save money too, but neither of these is its primary task, which is to hold together in one place otherwise incompatible accounts of disease.

Acknowledgements

This chapter is dedicated to all the multidisciplinary staff of the Whittington Hospital paediatric department with whom I worked for 35 years, in particular to the paediatricians Max Friedman (1931–1987) and Heather Mackinnon MBE, and the social worker Annie Souter (1953–2014) each of whose leadership made successful liaison possible. I am grateful to psychiatrists Andrew West and Lopa Winters for helpful comments on earlier drafts, and to the family who generously gave permission for me to use clinical material about them. Though I had cited Britton's third position many times in other contexts, I needed the child psychotherapist Dorothy Judd to show me its irresistible application to paediatric liaison.

Notes

[1] 'If the link between the parents perceived in love and hate can be tolerated in the child's mind it provides him with a prototype for an object relationship of a third kind in which he is a witness and not a participant. A third position then comes into existence from which object relationships can be observed. Given this, we can also envisage being observed. This provides us with a capacity for seeing ourselves in interaction with others and for entertaining another point of view whilst retaining our own, for reflecting on ourselves whilst being ourselves. I call the mental freedom provided by this process triangular space' (Britton, 1989).

[2] An experienced paediatrician reflects: '...asthma and migraine prove to be symptoms, not diseases; translations of the clinical history into medical shorthand. We are left to find out why this child experiences recurrent attacks of wheezing and that one recurrent headaches' (Smithells, 1982, p. 135).

[3] 'Paediatricians view childhood more positively than do child psychiatrists [who] rated their own parents as less caring than do paediatricians' (Lawrence and Adler, 1992, p. 82). Enzer et al. (1986) showed how psychiatrists see childhood as a time of struggle, powerlessness and conflict. In a more recent British study, Glazebrook et al. (2003) found that paediatricians missed the need for mental health attention in three-quarters of their patients whose SDQ (strengths and difficulties questionnaire) suggested they should have been referred.

[4] 'Although "medically unexplained" is scientifically neutral, it had surprisingly negative connotations for patients. Conversely, although doctors may think the term "functional" is pejorative, patients did not perceive it as such' (Stone et al., 2002). However, neurologists prefer the ambiguity of 'functional' (Kanaan et al., 2012).

[5] Campo and Fritz go on to give the following advice – a counsel of perfection – 'Given the pervasive nature of stigma, it is especially important to avoid communicating any sense of embarrassment regarding the diagnosis of somatoform disorder or other psychiatric disorder because this can contribute to treatment resistance and a patient's wish to perpetuate the search for traditional disease. Avoid mind–body dualism by discussing the relationship between mind and body and the false dichotomies presented by our current health care system' (Campo & Fritz, 2002, p. 470).

[6] Long before Western philosophy there was an understanding of mind–body unity, which still finds expression. Gregory Bateson (1979) follows a line of thinkers – from the ancient Egyptians and pre-Socratic philosophers to, in our time, Iain McGilchrist (2009) and others who see more continuity

between mind and matter. Descartes' contemporary Baruch Spinoza said *'Mind and body are one and the same thing'* (Spinoza, 1951, p. 131).

[7] 'While comparable brain changes were seen with both drug and placebo administration, drug response was not merely the same as the placebo effect' (Mayberg et al., 2002, p. 731).

[8] As in any setting a crucial quality of effective mental health intervention in paediatrics is the absence of blame. While family members may blame one another it is a clinical obligation not to take sides, but instead to make sense of the story. Therapists work hard at being 'non-judgemental'. 'This is not the absence of judgement, but the absence of blaming.' The psychoanalyst Wilfred Bion (1897–1979) spoke of the need to abandon 'memory and desire' (1970) when with a patient. Later Gianfranco Cecchin (1932–2004), one of the original Milan group of family systemic therapists, said one must be trained to achieve neutrality, 'to see the system, to be interested in it, to appreciate this kind of system without wanting to change it' (Boscolo et al., 1987, p. 152). From this position problems seem different already; they move from a fixed location to where they may be more easily observed by all players' (Kraemer, 2006, pp. 242–3). Where systematic lying or criminal abuse is part of the picture, non-blaming neutrality may have to be modified.

[9] *The James Spence Medal* is the highest honour in British paediatrics.

[10] Stone's study had a surprising outcome. Despite furious resistance from nurses in particular, a paediatric colleague opened one of his wards to unrestricted visiting while keeping the other limited to the usual minimal hours. Before any results could be obtained, within several months all the paediatric wards has opened their doors to parents (Karen, 1994, pp. 80–81).

[11] Leo Kanner wrote the first textbook of child psychiatry in the English language, published in 1935, and was the first to describe the syndrome of infantile autism.

[12] 'Sometimes, although the news came initially from doctors, ward staff would be left with the burden of dealing with the family's confusion or resistance: The family sits there nodding, but as the doctor goes away, then they sort of talk to the nurses and they automatically think it has been made up. They can't accept that the child has actually got psychological problems (Health Care Assistant)' (Furness et al., 2009, p. 580).

[13] '...the key features of quality consultation will remain unchanged. The consultant will continue to bring to the multidisciplinary medical team the combined expertise of psychodynamic understanding, psychopharmacology, a developmental perspective on the meaning of illness, adaptation to trauma, knowledge of psychiatric conditions, behavioural

interventions, and CNS influences in medical illnesses and as a result of medical treatment' (Pinsky et al., 2015, p. 596).

[14] 'Over 80% of paediatricians perceived access as a frequently encountered difficulty ... Paediatricians were frustrated with the current provision of consultations and some tried to manage by themselves as they did not expect any additional help from their local CAMHS.' (Slowik & Noronha, 2004). '...formalised liaison services were rare (provided by only one-third) and dedicated specialist CAMHS liaison services even rarer' (Woodgate and Garralda, 2006).

[15] While taking a more active part in the safeguarding of children in their care, no doubt due to a more urgent need to prevent harm, even death, befalling them.

[16] Kraemer, S. (unpublished) *National Guidance on Paediatric Mental Health Liaison* www.sebastiankraemer.com/docs/Kraemer%20National%20Guidance%20on%20Paediatric%20Mental%20Health%20Liaison.pdf

[17] 'One fifth of all children referred to local specialist NHS mental health services, are rejected for treatment' NSPCC, 12 October 2015 www.nspcc.org.uk/fighting-for-childhood/news-opinion/1-in-five-5-children-referred-to-local-mental-health-services-are-rejected-for-treatment/ (Accessed 10 February 2016).

[18] 'There has been a long and desultory flirtation between [paediatricians and child psychiatrists] but it is high time they were married – if only for the sake of the children' (paediatrician John Apley (1908–1980) cited by Hersov, 1986).

[19] Kanner could have added that sending a paediatric patient away to be treated elsewhere – such as CAMHS – is unlikely to appeal to the child and family unless they have already agreed that the primary problem is a mental or emotional one.

[20] 'Family therapy' is less off-putting.

[21] 'Having any physical complaint (compared with no physical health condition) increased the odds of having a mental disorder by 82%' (Meltzer et al., 2000).

[22] 'The estimated prevalence of a psychiatric diagnosis among children with reported chronic illness was 10%, almost twice the rate found in children without chronic illness' (Hysing et al., 2007).

[23] '...high levels of comorbid anxiety and to a lesser extent depressive disorders in childhood, functional somatic symptoms and somatoform disorders' (Garralda and Rask, 2015).

[24] Kraemer, S. (unpublished) *Paediatric psychology/mental health liaison: selected references www.sebastiankraemer.com/docs/Kraemer%20Liaisonrefs.pdf*

References

Abbass, A.A., Nowoweiski, S.J., Bernier, D., Tarzwell, R. and Beutel, M.E. (2014). Review of psychodynamic psychotherapy neuroimaging studies. Psychotherapy and Psychosomatics, 83 (3), 142–147.

A two year old goes to hospital: a scientific film. (1952). by James Robertson. [DVD] UK: Concord Media.

Bateson, G. (1979). *Mind and Nature: A Necessary Unity.* London: Wildwood House.

Bion, W.R. (1970). *Attention and Interpretation.* London: Tavistock Publications, p. 51.

Boscolo, L., Cecchin, G., Hoffman, L. and Penn, P. (1987). *Milan Systemic Therapy.* New York: Basic Books.

Brandon, S., Lindsay, M., Lovell-Davis, J. and Kraemer, S. (2009). 'What is wrong with emotional upset?' 50 years on from the Platt Report. *Archives of Disease in Childhood,* 94, 173–7.

Brenneman, J. (1931). The menace of psychiatry. *American Journal of Diseases of Children,* 42, 376–402, p. 391.

Britton, R. (1989). The missing link; parental sexuality in the Oedipus complex. In: R. Britton, M. Feldman and E. O'Shaughnessy (eds), *The Oedipus Complex Today: Clinical Implications.* London: Karnac, pp. 83–101.

Britton, R. (2015). *Between Mind and Brain.* London: Karnac.

Campo, J.V. and Fritz, G. (2001). A Management Model for Pediatric Somatization. *Psychosomatics,* 42, 467–476.

Carter, B. (2002). Chronic pain in childhood and the medical encounter: Professional ventriloquism and hidden voices. *Qualitative Health Research,* 12, 28–41.

Court, D. (1975). Sir James Spence. *Archives of Disease in Childhood,* 50, 85–9.

Davison, K. (2012). Autoimmunity in Psychiatry. *The British Journal of Psychiatry,* 200, 353–355.

Edwards, M. and Titman, P. (2010). *Promoting psychological well-being in children with acute and chronic illness.* London: Jessica Kingsley Publishers

Enzer, N.B., Singleton, D.S., Snellman L.A. et al. (1986). Interferences in collaboration between child psychiatrists and pediatricians: A fundamental difference in attitude toward childhood. *Journal of Developmental and Behavioral Pediatrics,* 7, 186–193.

Fivaz-Depeursinge, E., Cairo, S., Scaiola, C.L. and Favez, N. (2012). Nine-month-olds' triangular interactive strategies with their parents' couple in low-coordination families: A descriptive study. *Infant Mental Health Journal*, 33, 10–21.

Furness, P., Glazebrook, C., Tay, J., Abbas, K. and Slaveska-Hollis, K. (2009). Medically unexplained physical symptoms in children: exploring hospital staff perceptions. *Clinical Child Psychology and Psychiatry*, 14 (4), 575–587.

Garralda, M.E. and Rask, C. (2015). Somatoform and related disorders. In: A. Thapar, D.S. Pine, J.F. Leckman, S. Scott, M.J. Snowling and E. Taylor (eds), *Rutter's Child and Adolescent Psychiatry*, Chichester, UK: John Wiley and Sons, pp. 1035–1054, p. 1039.

Glazebrook, C., Hollis, C., Heussler, H., Goodman, R. and Coates, L. (2003). Detecting emotional and behavioural problems in paediatric clinics. *Child: Care, Health and Development*, 29, 141–149.

Hatcher, S. and Arroll, B. (2008). Assessment and management of medically unexplained symptoms. *British Medical Journal*, 336, 1124–1128.

Hersov, L. (1986). Child psychiatry in Britain – the last 30 years. *Journal of Child Psychology and Psychiatry*, 27, 781–801, p. 788.

Hinton, D. and Kirk, S. (2016). Families' and healthcare professionals' perceptions of healthcare services for children and young people with medically unexplained symptoms: a narrative review of the literature. *Health and Social Care in the Community*, 24, 12–16, p. 13.

Hrdy, S. B. (2016). Development plus social selection in the evolution of 'emotionally modern' humans. In: C.L. Meehan and A.N. Crittenden (eds), *Childhood: Origins, Evolution, and Implications*. Albuquerque NM: University of New Mexico Press, pp. 11–44.

Hysing, M., Elgen, I., Gillberg, G., Lie, S.A. and Lundervold, A.J. (2007). Chronic physical illness and mental health in children. Results from a large-scale population study. *Journal of Child Psychology and Psychiatry*, 48 (8), 785–92, p. 790.

Kanaan, R.A., Armstrong, D. and Wessely, S.C. (2012). The function of 'functional': A mixed methods investigation. *Journal of Neurology, Neurosurgery and Psychiatry*, 83 (3), 248–250.

Kanner, L. McKay, R.J. and Moody, E.E. (1953). Problems in Child Psychiatry. *Pediatrics*, 11, 393–404, p. 397.

Karen, R. (1994). *Becoming Attached*. Oxford: Oxford University Press, pp. 80–81.

Kennedy, I. (2010). *Getting it right for children and young people. Overcoming cultural barriers in the NHS so as to meet their needs.* London: Department of Health.

Kraemer, S. (2006). Something happens: elements of therapeutic change. *Clinical Child Psychology and Psychiatry*, 11, 239–48.

Kraemer, S. (2009). 'The menace of psychiatry': Does it still ring a bell? *Archives of Disease in Childhood,* 94(8), 570–572.

Kraemer, S. (2010). Liaison and co-operation between paediatrics and mental health. *Paediatrics and Child Health,* 20, 382–387, p. 384

Kraemer, S. (2015). Institutional blind spot around mental health needs of paediatric patients. [letter] *British Medical Journal,* 351, h3559.

Lancet (1952). The Young Child in Hospital [Annotation]. *Lancet* 260(6745), 1122–1123.

Lawrence, J. and Adler, R. (1992). Childhood through the eyes of child psychiatrists and paediatricians. *Australian and New Zealand Journal of Psychiatry,* 26 (1), 82–90.

Mayberg, H.S., Silva, J.A., Brannan, S.K., Tekell, J.L., Mahurin. R.K., McGinnis, S. and Jerabek, P.A. (2002). The functional neuroanatomy of the placebo effect. *American Journal of Psychiatry,* 159 (5), 728–37.

McGilchrist, I. (2009). *The Master and his Emissary.* Yale University Press.

Meltzer, H., Gatward, R., Goodman, R. and Ford, T. (2000). *Mental health of children and adolescents in Great Britain.* London: The Stationery Office, p. 74.

(The Platt Report) Ministry of Health, Central Health Services Council. (1959).*The Welfare of Children in Hospital: Report of the Committee.* London: HMSO.

Pinsky, E., Rauch, P. and Abrams A. (2015). Pediatric consultation and psychiatric aspects of somatic disease, In Thapar A, Pine D, Leckman, J. Scott S, Snowling, M., Taylor E *Rutter's Child and Adolescent Psychiatry.* Chichester, UK: Wiley.

Rask, C.U., Ørnbøl, E., Olsen, E.M., Fink, P. and Skovgaard, A.M. (2013). Infant behaviors are predictive of functional somatic symptoms at ages 5–7 years: Results from the Copenhagen Child Cohort CCC2000. *Journal of Pediatrics,* 162 (2), 335–342.

Robertson, J. and Robertson, J. (1989). *Separation and the Very Young.* London: Free Association Books.

Skirry, J. (2005). *Descartes and the Metaphysics of Human Nature.* London and New York: Thoemmes-Continuum Press.

Slowik, M. and Noronha, S. (2004). Need for child mental health consultation and paediatricians' perception of these services. *Child and Adolescent Mental Health,* 9, 121–4.

Smithells, R.W. (1982). In praise of outpatients: partnerships in paediatrics. In J. Apley and C. Ounsted, *One Child, Clinics in Developmental Medicine no. 80.* London: SIMP, pp. 135–46.

Spence, J.C. (1947). The care of children in hospital. *British Medical Journal* 1(4490), 125–130.

Spence, S.A. (2006). All in the mind? The neural correlates of unexplained physical symptoms. *Advances in Psychiatric Treatment,* 12, 349–358.

Spinoza, B. (1951). *The Chief Works of Benedict de Spinoza, vol 2.* R.H.M. Elwes, trans. New York: Dover, p. 131.

Stone, J., Wojcik, W., Durrance, D. et al. (2002). What should we say to patients with symptoms unexplained by disease? The 'number needed to offend'. *British Medical Journal*, 325, 1449–50.

Tennant, C. and McLean, L. (2001). The impact of emotions on coronary heart disease risk. *Journal of Cardiovascular Risk*, 8 (3), 175–183.

White, P.D., Rickards, H. and Zeman, A.Z. (2012). Time to end the distinction between mental and neurological illnesses. *British Medical Journal*, 344, e3454.

Woodgate, M. and Garralda, M. (2006). Paediatric liaison work by child and adolescent mental health services. *Child and Adolescent Mental Health*, 11, 19–24.

Wright, J. and Potter, P. (eds) (2000). *Psyche and Soma, physicians and metaphysicians on the mind-body problem from antiquity to enlightenment*. Oxford: Oxford University Press, p. 4.

6

THE WIDER CLINICAL AND SOCIAL CONTEXT OF ADHD

Louise Richards

Ever since the dawn of culture ethics has been an essential part of the heal-ing art. Conflicting loyalties for physicians in contemporary society, the deli-cate nature of the therapist-patient relationship, and the possibility of abuses of psychiatric concepts, knowledge and technology in actions contrary to the laws of humanity, all make high ethical standards more necessary than ever for those practicing the art and science of psychiatry. (World Psychiatric Association: The Declaration of Hawaii 1977)

As a UK Child and Adolescent Psychiatrist, the construct of ADHD has presented more ethical dilemmas than any other facet of my clinical practice. It was the experience of arriving as a new con-sultant to a large caseload of young people treated with stimulant medication within a largely biological framework which particularly alarmed me though, and prompted my interest in psychosocial fac-tors linked to ADHD.

My concerns were twofold:

1. The frequency with which 'on scratching the surface' it became evident that many of these young people were struggling with internal and external factors related to their family and wider environment. Conceptualising ADHD symptoms within a pre-dominantly biological aetiological model had meant that poten-tially serious disturbances in familial attachments or safeguarding concerns were being overlooked or minimised, and the associated psychological sequelae left effectively untreated. At the other extreme, stimulant medication was being prescribed potentially for many years, in situations where a relatively brief psychologi-cal or systemic intervention may well have sufficed.

2. It was very unclear whether young people had been involved in the decision making around medication being prescribed for them. This was despite the relatively high prevalence of side-effects associated with stimulant medication use, including over-sedation, particularly at higher doses. I also had considerable ethical misgivings about prescribing for a child, before they were of an age or developmental stage to be able to give informed consent or even articulate possible side-effects.

Attention deficit/hyperactivity disorder (ADHD) has been described as 'among the most frequent, intensely researched, and yet diagnostically controversial conditions of childhood' (Dwivedi Banhatti 2005). Few would debate the existence of a group of children/adolescents who struggle with the classic triad of ADHD symptoms: hyperactivity, impulsivity and inattention. However, many have argued that the current dominant ADHD construct is overly simplistic and privileges biological aetiological factors and treatment modalities (particularly medication), while neglecting a more holistic understanding and treatment approach:

> Once the problem is located in the child, the field of intervention narrows, since the aim is to dispose of the problem rather than to understand it. (McFadyen, 1997)

> When children express difficult behavior this often communicates that all is not well in the child's life...a rapid rush to an ADHD diagnosis because of parental pressure, limited mental health and welfare resources and lack of time can result in deeper problems being overlooked. (Jureidini, 2001)

Concurrently while the evidence as to the long-term efficacy of stimulant medication has remained at best poor (Jensen et al., 2007; Parens and Johnson, 2011, S16-17), and that of the potential long-term side-effects (including the impact on neural pathways) uncertain, the use of medication to treat ADHD has continued to rise exponentially globally (e.g. Scheffler et al., 2007). With sales estimated to reach record levels by 2018 (Global Data 2011), and unprecedented prevalence rates of medication use in the United States one might think this was a matter for celebrating amongst those original proponents of ADHD. Instead Professor Conners (whose questionnaire remains a central component of diagnosis of ADHD) has been reported as questioning the rising rates of diagnosis, calling them 'a national disaster of dangerous proportions' and a '..concoction to justify the giving out of medication at unprecedented and unjustifiable levels' (Schwarz 2013)

The DSM (Diagnostic and Statistical Manual of Mental Disorders) position on behavioural disorders has been criticised as having contributed to this reductionist ethic by encouraging a tick-box approach to procuring a diagnosis of ADHD with the 'emphasis (being) on listing symptoms rather than listening to what the families might be able to tell us about themselves' (Jureidini 2009). The subjective nature of this approach has also been equally frequently alluded to as a concern (e.g. Schmidt Neven, Anderson and Godber 2002a) but could have been no better highlighted than the findings of the recent Great Smoky Mountain longitudinal study which suggested that 7.3% of the 1,422 children studied had received stimulants at some time during the four-year study period. However, when the researchers compared their application of DSM criteria to these children, their reported conclusion was that there had been 'overdiagnosis, misdiagnosis and underdiagnosis (of ADHD)', and that '...more children without ADHD received stimulants than did children with ADHD' (Parens and Johnston, 2011 S15).

Critics of DSM by no means belong to the minority, as the ex-Chair of DSMIV Frances Allen has himself recurrently expressed concern about the harmful unintended consequences of DSM as having contributed to psychiatric fads, diagnostic inflation and over medication (e.g. Frances 2011) particularly in the context of aggressive marketing by the pharmaceutical drug industry with attention deficit disorder given as a specific example of this:

> Drug companies were given the means, the motive, and the message to disease-monger ADHD and blow it up out of all proportion. They succeeded beyond all expectations in achieving a triumph of clever advertising over common sense. (Frances 2014)

While many have written about the pervasive influence of the pharmaceutical drug industry including professional conflicts of interests, links with DSM, ADHD Parent Support Groups and the impact of Direct-to-Consumer-Advertising within the United States, the details remain disturbing (e.g. Schwarz, 2013; Furman, 2009; Timimi, 2009). Leo and Lacasse (2009) used the example of the Adderrall 2005 advertising campaign to illustrate the degree to which these adverts overly inflated the positive benefits of medication, linking these with understandable and universal fears parents might have about their children, while minimising the potential side effects of Adderall.

It is commonly accepted though that beyond the impact of the pharmaceutical drug industry, the reasons underlying the widely discrepant international, and interstate ADHD diagnostic and medication rates are highly complex and multifactorial:

> A number of social and economic forces heavily influence the creation and use of diagnostic categories and decisions about which treatments are used. These forces help to explain why many children do not receive careful diagnoses, why evidence-based treatments are often not available, and why promising changes to children's environments are not made.' (Parens-Johnston 2011 S20)

The US report (quoted above) summarised the findings of a series of workshops involving clinicians, researchers, scholars and advocates from a variety of disciplinary backgrounds, which had sought to understand the diagnostic controversies and reasons for the rising medication use in relation to ADHD. It gives a unique and arguably troubling insight into ADHD treatment within the United States, highlighting amongst other concerns the impact of the US health care system and its associated economic pressures. By encouraging brief and infrequent treatment appointments; limiting the availability of psychosocial interventions and opportunities for interagency liaison; and undermining the quality of clinician training, managed care was postulated to increase the likelihood of diagnostic mistakes, and that psychotropic medication alone would be the default treatment (S23–25). L. Diller (paediatrician) concurrently highlighted the impact of a stretched educational system, and the ethical concerns associated with the tendency for teachers and schools to promote medication interventions in the face of pressure to perform with decreased funding, increased classroom sizes and fewer educational supports. Learning disorders were said to be frequently undiagnosed and untreated, as medication was prescribed in the absence of a developmental or educational assessment. 'Our educational institutions along with the mental health delivery system foster a bias towards medication in the classroom over practices that engage the child but potentially cost more money and time.' (S21)

Hinshaw and Scheffler (2014) sought to analyse the reasons underlying the hugely discrepant ADHD diagnostic rates in youth aged 4 to 17 (in 2007) shown in North Carolina to be 15.5% (of which 74.4% were medicated) and 6% in California (of which 49% were medicated). They concluded the most likely explanatory factors to be:

1. The impact of DTCA advertisement of which the South was reported to have the highest number of subscriptions.

2. The discrepant introduction across the United States of educational policies implemented to encourage teachers and schools to improve educational quality by providing incentives (including financial rewards for enhanced performance) and sanctions (for lack of gains); but said to have had the unintended consequence of increasing ADHD diagnostic rates.

Within the United Kingdom, as prescriptions for Ritalin were reported to quadruple in the decade preceding 2010, concern was expressed about rising psycho-stimulant medication use including in preschoolers (e.g. Doward and Craig, 2012). However, while 6.1% of children in the United States are reported to receive drugs for ADHD, this compared with an estimated 0.8% in the United Kingdom (McCarthy et al., 2012). In the United Kingdom, NICE Guidelines (2009) advise parenting programmes and alternative educational support as first-line interventions in all but severe presentations. Moreover, in contrast to the United States where preschoolers aged 3–5.5 years have been enrolled in medication trials for the treatment of ADHD (e.g. Kollins et al., 2006), medication use in preschoolers is not generally advised by NICE (2009).

Returning to my arrival as a new consultant, I faced a group of children being treated for ADHD symptoms within a largely biological framework, while my direct clinical experience revealed a diversity of psychosocial factors. Two clinical groups particularly exemplified this 'disconnect':

1. Those young people attending schools for emotional and behaviourally disturbed children and adolescents of which up to 70% have been shown to have ADHD (Cassidy, James, and Wiggs, 2001; Place et al., 2000). This is a group acknowledged to have multi-complex difficulties including their home

circumstances, unsettled relationships, difficulties with siblings, experience of traumatic events, substance abuse, sometimes criminal involvement; and chronic emotional challenges where perhaps 25% of pupils in special schools for young people exhibiting emotional and behavioural disturbances (EBD) have been, or are, looked after (Cole et al., 2002).

2. Looked after children – a group we know to have experienced high rates of abuse, trauma, losses, attachment deficits and anxiety – and amongst whom the prevalence of ADHD (and other disorders) is recorded to be 5–7 times that seen in private household children (Meltzer et al., 2002).

In addition, clinical experience, coupled with a literature review (Richards 2013) revealed a group of children who were particularly appropriate for therapeutic input as an effective alternative to stimulant medication. About a quarter to one-third of children with ADHD were said to also meet criteria for anxiety disorder. This group of children had also been found to experience more stressful life events, such as divorce and separation, than those who present with ADHD alone (Pliszka, 2000).

I had been fortunate that my clinical training had incorporated exposure to a range of therapeutic modalities and treatment approaches within child mental health. My experience in adult psychiatry proved similarly helpful. With the support of multi-disciplinary team colleagues we developed a more holistic therapeutic approach, where ADHD symptoms had been seen previously as largely the responsibility of the child psychiatrist. The range of therapeutic interventions used included interagency liaison, family therapy, parent support, individual work with the child/adolescent, and parent–child work (particularly in the event of attachment concerns). When used, stimulant medication tended to be at the lowest efficacious dose, for the minimum time necessary, and very much informed by feedback from the young person as to how they perceived the relative side-effect/benefits. Adjunctive therapeutic approaches meant that several young people were enabled to manage at reduced doses, or even medication-free. Concurrent school support, or indeed alternative placements where indicated, was stressed, as was the importance of education psychology assessments.

As I sought to understand the 'disconnect' previously described, I was struck by an earlier study which had shown that being told that a child had a diagnosis of ADHD made clinicians less likely to notice psychosocial issues and family factors impacting on that child, and even to ask about physical abuse:

Overmeyer, Taylor, Blanz and Schmidt (1999), comparing 21 hyperkinetic and 26 conduct disordered children, had shown that while blind raters found a similar frequency of psychosocial adversities in both groups, clinical raters who knew the diagnosis of the children rated adverse psychosocial situations as much lower in hyperkinetic children than in children with conduct disorder. This effect was particularly pronounced in the area of abnormal intrafamilial relationships: lack of warmth in parent–child relationship; hostility or scapegoating of child and intrafamilial discord amongst adults. Blind raters routinely asked about physical abuse, but clinical raters did not.

It seemed therefore as if the pendulum had shifted in how children's difficult or troubling behaviour was framed, explained and managed. Previously psychosocial explanations had tended to accompany such labels as 'emotional and behavioural disorders' (educational), and 'oppositional defiant or conduct disorders' (medical), with the attendant risk of a parental blame culture. With the emergence of ADHD as a global phenomenon and the rapid associated medication use, biological aetiologies now predominated, with the danger of now neglecting psychosocial factors that might be contributing to children's behaviour. Concurrently, there had arisen a tendency to oversimplify the interrelationship between ADHD and conduct disorder symptoms. Thus while the dominant discourse counselled that treating ADHD symptoms with stimulant medication was necessary to avert conduct disorder amongst other possible negative sequelae (e.g. Coghill 2005); others argued that the adjunctive symptoms of conduct disorder were a result of parental/family factors which might equally be exacerbating ADHD symptoms in a young person. Sroufe argued that:

> When maladaption is viewed as a development rather than a disease, a transformed understanding results and a fundamentally different research agenda emerges. Within a developmental perspective, maladaption is viewed as evolving through the successive adaptions of persons in their environments. It is not something a person 'has' or an ineluctable expression of an endogenous pathogen. It is the complex result of a myriad of risk and protective factors operating over time. (Sroufe, 1997, p. 1)

ADHD and conduct disorder was said to co-occur in 30–50% of cases in both epidemiological and clinical samples (Biederman, Newcorn and Sprich, 1991, cited in Biederman, Faraone and Kiely, 1996); and to be a group known prognostically to have poorer outcomes in terms of greater risk of aggressive and delinquent behaviour, as well as school dysfunction, than ADHD alone. Concurrently while there was a generally accepted association between parental psychopathology and comorbid ADHD-oppositional disorder/conduct disorder in their children (including maternal depression and borderline personality disorder; and parental anti-social personality disorder, alcoholism and substance use) (see Review: Richards, 2013) there seemed to be a tendency to focus on biological causal links for this. Hence it was suggested that ADHD and comorbid conduct disorder might represent a separate familial subtype given the high rate of anti-social disorders amongst first-degree relatives of children sharing both diagnoses. ADHD and depression were also proposed to share familial vulnerabilities (Thapar et al., 1999).

What seemed barely acknowledged though was the part parent–child relational, or indeed shared environmental, factors might have played in potentially contributing to the poor prognostic factors and attendant aggression and delinquency seen within this group. This was despite the fact that parental alcohol abuse and personality disorders are recognised risk factors for child abuse, especially where there is associated parental violence (Duncan and Reder, 2000; Drummond and Fitzpatrick, 2000; Westman, 2000). Children living in such families are known to be at greater risk of trauma, whether to themselves, or in witnessing inter-parental violence, or maternal self-harm (in the case of mothers with a diagnosis of borderline personality disorder). Neglect is another possibility. Emotional abuse and neglect have also been highlighted as perhaps the most relevant and problematic types of maltreatment associated with parental mental illness. In many cases, the neglect of their children's emotional needs may be unintentional, but damaging effects on children's development still occurs (Royal College of Psychiatrists, 2002).

Moreover, several studies had shown high rates of ADHD amongst children who have been maltreated (e.g. Merry, Franz and Andrews, 1994; McCleer et al. 1994). High rates of abuse (including physical, sexual and neglect) had concurrently been found amongst children with ADHD (e.g. Briscoe-Smith and Hinshaw 2006

Ouyang et al. 2008). Interactional effects of trauma had also been shown: Cohen et al. (2002) found that parental marital disruption when combined with a history of physical abuse increased the risk of lifetime ADHD 15-fold (compared with non-abused adolescents from intact families). Exposure to domestic violence, particularly when combined with physical abuse, had also been associated with higher rates of a lifetime diagnosis of ADHD (Pelcovitz et al., 2000). Indeed Chiodo et al. (2008) in their study regarding the impact of family violence on children seen in a children's aid society showed that virtually a third of the group of children who had both witnessed domestic violence and experienced physical abuse were deemed diagnosable with ADHD.

Amongst children with ADHD, co-existing oppositional/conduct disorder and higher rates of externalising behaviours and peer rejection have been shown to characterise those who have been abused. (Briscoe-Smith and Hinshaw 2006; Ford et al., 1999). However, in studies of maltreated children, considerable comorbidity has been found between PTSD, ADHD and oppositional defiant disorder, raising the question whether those symptoms resulting in the diagnosis of ADHD and oppositional disorder actually reflects anxiety associated with PTSD secondary to their maltreatment (e.g. McLeer et al., 1994; Famularo, Kinscherff and Fenton, 1992).

Clearly it is not the case that all children presenting with ADHD symptoms will have experienced maltreatment. However, this possibility does need to be considered as part of a holistic assessment, and also where a child being treated for ADHD presents with a deterioration or change in their presentation. Equally, if a child has had abusive experiences, an integrated broadly psychotherapeutic approach will generally be needed, including attention to traumatic sequelae.

There is a much broader issue highlighted here though, which many parents and clinicians take seriously when weighing up the pros and cons of prescribing stimulant medication for an individual child. The current accepted wisdom is that we need to treat ADHD medically to avoid a range of negative sequelae (e.g. Coghill 2005). To take one example though, De Sanctis et al. (2008) found that in the absence of maltreatment and/or comorbid conduct disorder, children with ADHD were at no greater risk for substance-use disorders than the general population. Far more longitudinal research is needed therefore to elucidate whether these adverse outcomes are mediated via psychosocial factors. Otherwise it may well be the case that a significant number of children and adolescents are being prescribed stimulant medication for ADHD symptoms, which though challenging for parents and schools to manage in the short term are not necessarily of long-term significance.

McArdle, O'Brien and Kolvin (1995) amply demonstrated this in their longitudinal study involving 3,300 11 and 12-year-old senior school children, and 1,040 and year-old children (52% M and 48% F) in Newcastle, UK which sought to address the question whether hyperactivity was a risk factor for conduct disorder. Their ultimate conclusion was that: 'a crucial finding is that whereas 28.4% of the junior school children with hyperactivity were conduct disordered, the rate of conduct disorder amongst senior school children with hyperactivity was less than half that (12.9%). This suggests that the extent of the link with conduct disorders appears, in fact, to decline with age, and further, that some forms of hyperactivity, home based especially, may have few current or longitudinal implications.'

A significant association has also been found between maternal depression and comorbid ADHD and oppositional/conduct disorder in their child. Possible explanations for this include: maternal mental states biasing the mother's perception, shared genetics and external factors, and children developing emotional or behavioural problems in reaction to their mother's distress or disturbances in parenting style. Depression may result in mothers being less emotionally available, and more critical and negative about their children (Hibbs et al., 1991, cited in Woodward et al., 1998). Equally, caring for a child with problematic behavior can lead to, or exacerbate, maternal depression. Child conduct problems, maternal depressive symptoms and maternal responsiveness have been hypothesised to be linked in a reciprocal and transactional fashion, with each component influencing the development of each other component over time (Johnson et al., 2002).

A separate though connected issue is whether treating parents may sometimes have a larger effect on outcome than treating the index child. A fascinating study by Modell et al. (2001) followed up 24 mothers recently diagnosed with major depressive disorder, and showed the benefits which followed one–two months' treatment with an antidepressant in that maternal ratings of their children's behaviour significantly improved, with improved scores in conduct, learning problems and impulsive-hyperactive sub-scales accounting for 89% of this reported behavioural change. The degree of reported improvement was highly correlated with the degree of improvement in depressive symptoms.

If parental mental illness and other aspects of family dysfunction are not acknowledged, or treated, then viewing a child's ADHD symptoms as an individual problem is unlikely to be successful. Mental health professionals are well placed to sensitively explore symptoms suggestive of mental illness in parents and liaise with general practitioners and adult mental health services to access appropriate support where necessary. Such families may well benefit from family therapy (Lange et al., 2005) or a therapeutic intervention addressing the parent–child relationship particularly if there are signs of an insecure attachment. Moreover, in families where there are possible child protection concerns, a very different 'therapeutic' approach will be needed that 'treats' their symptoms within a systemic framework with multi-agency input, including social services and adult mental health services.

This brings me finally to the Multimodal Treatment Study of Children with ADHD (MTA, 1999): a 14-month, multisite, randomised clinical trial undertaken in the United States (1994–1998) involving 576 boys and girls (aged 7–9 years), the results of which influenced treatment regimes for ADHD globally, leading to the mainstay of recommended treatment for ADHD being stimulant medication and behavioural treatment. Concern has been expressed though that with insecurely attached children, such approaches might fail to address the underlying problem (Clarke et al., 2002), and leave children who are frustrated and anxious over the lack of a parental bond 'feeling more victimized' (Erdman, 1998, p. 183). Moreover, several have questioned how generaliseable its findings are, postulating that its burdensome requirements limited enlistment to motivated families in supportive schools who differed considerably from families usually referred to child mental health settings (e.g. Boyle and Jahad, 1999). Leslie et al. (2006) illustrated this, comparing two groups from a community and private office in San Diego with similar rates of ADHD. Children in community clinics were more likely to have experienced foster care, child abuse and/or neglect, homelessness, parental drug use and witnessed domestic violence; to have at least one other family member (usually a parent) with a mental disorder; and to screen positively for oppositional/ conduct disorder.

An additional issue (evidenced by neurobiological and attachment research) is that while genetic predisposition is a fixed variable, psychosocial factors can be additive in their impacts and modulated over the course of a young person's development either positively or deleteriously (Richards 2013). The impact of maltreatment, traumatic experiences and/or exposure to parental psychopathology will differ considerably depending on the child's age and developmental stage. Family life can also vary longitudinally for a multiplicity of reasons, including difficult financial and emotional/social circumstances, and with that the capacity for parents to manage their children's behaviour. Conceptualising the aetiology of ADHD symptoms in these terms has important implications in influencing how one approaches the subsequent treatment plan.

To conclude, I hope this chapter has demonstrated some of the complexities and controversies accompanying the ADHD construct and the acknowledged escalating use of stimulant medication. If we as a global community are to properly grapple with the associated clinical and social ethical considerations, then a far more integrated and sophisticated approach will be needed at both clinical and policy level.

References

Biederman, J., Faraone, S. and Kiely, K. (1996). Comorbidity in outcome of attention-deficit/hyperactivity disorder. In L. Hechtman (ed.), *Do they grow out of it? Long-term outcomes of childhood disorders*. Washington, USA and London, UK: American Psychiatric Press.

Biederman, J., Newcorn, J. and Sprich, S. (1991). Comorbidity of attention deficit hyperactivity disorder with conduct, depressive, anxiety and other disorders. *The American Journal of Psychiatry*, 148, 564–577.

Boyle, M. and Jahad, R. (1999). Lessons from large trials: The MTA Study as a model for evaluating the treatment of childhood psychiatric disorder. *The Canadian Journal of Psychiatry*, 44, 991–998.

Briscoe-Smith, A. and Hinshaw, S. (2006). Linkages between child abuse and attention-deficit/hyperactivity disorder in girls: Behavioural and social correlates. *Child Abuse and Neglect* 30 1239–1255.

Cassidy, E., James, A. and Wiggs, L. (2001). The prevalence of psychiatric disorder in children attending a school for pupils with emotional and behavioural difficulties. *British Journal of Special Education*, 28 (4), 167–173.

Chiodo, D., Leschied, A., Whitehead, P. and Hurley, D. (2003). *The impact of violence on child outcomes in a child protection sample: implications for intervention*. Research Project: The University of Western Ontario.

Clarke, L., Ungerer, J. and Chahoud, K. (2002). Attachment Deficit Hyperactivity Disorder is associated with attachment insecurity. *Clinical Child Psychology and Psychiatry*, 7 (2), 179–198.

Coghill, D. (2005). Attention-deficit hyperactivity disorder: Should we believe the mass media or peer-reviewed literature? *Psychiatric Bulletin*, 29, 288–291.

Cohen, A., Adler, N., Kaplan, S., Pelcovitz, D. and Mandel, F. (2002) Interactional effects of marital status and physical abuse on adolescent psychopathology. *Child Abuse and Neglect*, 26, 277–288.

Cole, T., Selman, E., Daniels, H. and Visser, D. (2002). *The mental health needs of young people with emotional and behavioural difficulties*. Report Commissioned by the Mental Health Foundation, UK.

De Sanctis, V.A., Trampush, J.W., Marks, D.J., Miller, C.J., Harty, S.C., Newcorn, J.H. and Halperin, J.M. (2008). Childhood maltreatment and conduct disorder: Independent predictors of adolescent substance use disorders in youth with ADHD. *Journal of Clinical Child and Adolescent Psychology*, 37 (4), 785–793.

Doward, J. and Craig, E. (6 May 2012). Ritalin use for ADHD children soars fourfold. *The Guardian*. UK.

Drummond, C. and Fitzpatrick, G. (2000). Children of substance-misusing parents. In P. Reder, M. McClure and A. Jolley (eds), *Family Matters: Interfaces between Child and Adult Mental Health* (pp. 135–149). London and Philadelphia: Routledge.

Duncan, S. and Reder, P. (2000). Children's experience of major psychiatric disorder in their parent: An over view. In P. Reder, M. McClure and A. Jolley (eds), *Family Matters: Interfaces between Child and Adult Mental Health* (pp. 83–95). London and Philadelphia: Routledge.

Dwivedi, K.N. and Banhatti, R. G. (2005) Attention deficit/hyperactivity disorder and ethnicity. *Arch Dis Child, 90 Suppl* 1:i10–12.

Erdman, P. (1998). Conceptualising ADHD as a contextual response to parental attachment. *The American Journal of Family Therapy*, 26 (2), 177–185.

Famularo, R., Kinscherff, R. and Fenton, T. (1992). Psychiatric diagnosis of maltreated children: Preliminary findings. *Journal of the American Academy of Child and Adolescent Psychiatry*, 31, 863–867.

Ford, J.D., Racusin, R., Daviss, W.B., Ellis, C.G., Thomas, J., Rogers, K. and Sengupta, A. (1999). Trauma exposure among children with oppositional defiant disorder and attention deficit-hyperactivity disorder. *Journal of Consulting and Clinical Psychology*, 67 (5), 786–789.

Frances, A. Attention Deficit Disorder Epidemic: Real or Fad. Posted Online May 2011. *DSM5 in Distress. Psychology Today*.

Frances, A. How parents can protect kids from the ADHD 'epidemic'. Posted Online 2nd December 2014. *The Blog. Huffington Post.*

Furman, L. (2009). ADHD: What do we really know? In S. Timimi and J. Leo (eds), *Rethinking ADHD* (pp. 21–57). USA and UK: Palgrave Macmillan.

Global Data (2011). Published Report: Attention Deficit Hyperactivity Disorder (ADHD) Therapeutics – Pipeline Assessment and Market Forecasts to 2018. Summary published online.

Hibbs, E., Hamburger, S., Leane, M., Rapoport, J., Kruesi, M., Keysor, C. and Goldstein, M. (1991). Determinants of expressed emotion in families of disturbed and normal children. *Journal of Child Psychology and Psychiatry*, 32, 757–770.

Hinshaw, S.P. and Scheffler, R.M. (eds) *The ADHD Explosion: Myths, Medication, Money and Today's Push for Performance.* USA: Oxford University Press.

Jensen, P.S., Arnold, L.E., Swanson, J.M., Vitiello, B., Abikoff, H.B., Greenhill, L.L. and Hur, K. (2007). 3-year follow-up of the NIMH MTA study. *Journal of the American Academy of Child and Adolescent Psychiatry*, 46 (8), 989–1002.

Johnston, C., Murray, C., Hinshaw, S., Pelham, W. and Hoza, B. (2002). Responsiveness in interactions of mothers and sons with ADHD: Relations to maternal and child characteristics. *Journal of Abnormal Child Psychology*, 30 (1), 77–89.

Jureidini, J. (2001). Kids and Drugs (article by Carmel Sparke). *HQ,* 80, March, pp. 90–5. Cited in Schmidt Neven, R., Anderson, V., and Godber, T. (2002b). A critique of the medical model. In R.S. Neven, V. Anderson and T. Godber (eds), *Rethinking ADHD: Integrated Approaches to Helping Children at Home and at School* (pp. 39–57). Australia: Allen and Unwin Press.

Jureidini, J. (2009). Mind Magic. In S. Timimi and J. Leo (eds), *Rethinking ADHD* (pp. 349–359). USA and UK: Palgrave Macmillan.

Kollins, S. et al. (2006). Rationale, design, and methods of the Preschool ADHD Treatment Study (PATS). *Journal of American Academy of Child and Adolescent Psychiatry* 45 (11) 1275–83.

Lange, G., Sheerin, D., Carr, A., Dooley, B., Barton, V., Marshall, D. and Doyle, M. (2005). Family factors associated with attention deficit hyperactivity disorder and emotional disorders in children. *Journal of Family Therapy*, 27, 76–96.

Leslie, L., Stallone, K., Weckerly, J., McDaniel, A. and Monn, A. (2006). Implementing ADHD guidelines in primary care: Does one size fit all? *Journal of Health Care for the Poor and Underserved*, 17 (2), 302–327.

Leo, J. and Lacasse, J. (2009). The manipulation of data and attitudes about ADHD: A study of consumer advertisements. In S. Timimi and J. Leo (eds), *Rethinking ADHD* (pp. 133–159). USA and UK: Palgrave Macmillan.

McCarthy, S., Wilton, L., Murray, M.L. et al. (2012). The epidemiology of pharmacologically treated attention deficit hyperactivity disorder (ADHD) in children, adolescents and adults in UK primary care. *BMC Pediatr.* 12:78. (cited by Childhood attention-deficit disorder *BMJ* 2015;350:h2168.

McArdle, P., O'Brien, G. and Kolvin, I. (1995). Hyperactivity: Prevalence and relationship with conduct disorder. *Journal of Child Psychology and Psychiatry*, 36 (2), 279–303.

McFadyen, A. (1997). Reactivity or hyperactivity. Putting ADHD in a developmental and social context. Talk given at Tavistock Clinic, London. Cited in: Schmidt Neven, R., Anderson, V., and Godber, T. (2002b). A critique of the medical model. In R.S. Neven, V. Anderson and T. Godber (eds), *Rethinking ADHD: Integrated Approaches to Helping Children at Home and at School* (pp. 39–57). Australia: Allen and Unwin Press.

McLeer, S., Callaghan, M., Henry, D. and Wallen, J. (1994). Psychiatric disorders in sexually abused children. *Journal of the American Academy of Child and Adolescent Psychiatry*, 3 (3), 313–319.

Meltzer, H., Gatward, R., Corbin, T., Goodman, R. and Ford, T. *The Mental Health of Young People Looked After by Local Authorities in England.* The Report of a Survey carried out in 2002 by Social Survey Division for National Statistics on behalf of the Department of Health.

Merry, S., Franz, C.P. and Andrews, L. (1994). Psychiatric status of sexually abused children 12 months after disclosure of abuse. *Journal of the American Academy of Child and Adolescent Psychiatry*, 33 (7), 939–944.

Modell, J., Modell, J., Wallander, J., Hodgens, B., Duke, L. and Wisely, D. (2001). Maternal ratings of child behavior improve with treatment of maternal depression. *Family Medicine*, 3 (9), 691–695.

(The) NICE Guideline on diagnosis and management of ADHD in children, young people and adults. (2009). *National Clinical Practice Guideline Number 72.* England: The British Psychological Society and The Royal College of Psychiatrists.

Ouyang, L., Fang, X., Mercy, J., Perou, R. and Grosse, S. (2008). Attention-deficit/hyperactivity disorder symptoms and child maltreatment: A population-based study. *The Journal of Paediatrics*, 153, 851–856.

Overmeyer, S., Taylor, E., Blanz, B. and Schmidt, M.H. (1999). Psychosocial adversities underestimated in hyperkinetic children. *Journal of Child Psychology and Psychiatry*, 40 (2), 259–263.

Parens, E. and Johnson, J. (March-April 2011) *Troubled Children: Diagnosing, Treating, and Attending to Context.* Hastings Center Special Report.

Pelcovitz, D., Kaplan, S.J., De Rosa, R.R., Mandel, F.S. and Salzinger, S. (2000). Psychiatric disorders in adolescents exposed to domestic violence and physical abuse. *American Journal of Orthopsychiatry*, 70 (3), 360–369.

Place, M., Wilson, J., Martin, E. and Hulsmeier, J. (2000). The frequency of emotional and behavioural disturbance in an EBD school. *Child Psychology and Psychiatry Review*, 5 (2), 76–80.

Pliszka, S. (2000). Patterns of psychiatric comorbidity with attention-deficit/ hyperactivity disorder. *Child and Adolescent Psychiatric Clinics of North America*, 9, 525–540.

Richards, L.M.E. (2013). It is time for a more integrated bio-psycho-social approach to ADHD. *Clin Child Psychol Psychiatry*, 18 (4), 483–503.

Royal College of Psychiatrists. (2002). *Patients as parents: addressing the needs, including the safety of children whose parents have mental illness.* Council Report CR105.

Scheffler, R.M., Hinshaw, S.P., Modrek, S. and Levine, P. (2007). The global market for ADHD medications. *Health Affairs*, 26 (2), 450–457.

Schmidt Neven, R., Anderson, V. and Godber, T. (2002a). Neuropsychology and the diagnostic dilemmas of ADHD. In R.S. Neven, V. Anderson and T. Godber (eds), *Rethinking ADHD: Integrated Approaches to Helping Children at Home and at School* (pp. 14–38). Australia: Allen and Unwin Press.

Schmidt Neven, R., Anderson, V. and Godber, T. (2002b). A critique of the medical model. In R.S. Neven, V. Anderson and T. Godber (eds), *Rethinking ADHD: Integrated Approaches to Helping Children at Home and at School* (pp. 39–57). Australia: Allen and Unwin Press.

Schwarz, A. (December 2013). The Selling of Attention Deficit Disorder. *New York Times* published online.

Sroufe, A. (1997). Psychopathology as an outcome of development. *Development and Psychopathology*, 9, 251–268.

Thapar, A., Holmes, J., Poulton, K. and Harrington, R. (1999). Genetic basis of attention deficit and hyperac- tivity. *British Journal of Psychiatry*, 174, 105–111.

The MTA Cooperative Group. (1999). A 14-month randomized clinical trial of treatment strategies for attention-deficit/hyperactive disorder. *Archives of General Psychiatry*, 56, 1073–1086.

Timimi, S. (2009). Why diagnosis of ADHD has increased so rapidly in the West: A cultural perspective. In S. Timimi and J. Leo (eds), *Rethinking ADHD* (pp. 133–159). USA and UK: Palgrave Macmillan.

Westman, A. (2000). The problem of parental personality. In P. Reder, M. McClure and A. Jolley (eds), *Family Matters: Interfaces between Child and Adult Mental Health* (pp. 150–165). London and Philadelphia: Routledge.

Woodward, L., Taylor, E. and Downdey, L. (1998). The parenting and family functioning of children with hyperactivity. *Journal of Child Psychology and Psychiatry*, 39 (2), 161–169.

7

CULTURAL CONTEXT AND SOCIALLY INCLUSIVE PRACTICE

Steven Walker

Introduction

This chapter looks at the different ways culture is thought about and represented externally and internally in modern society and in the ways children and young people perceive themselves. Children's service providers are faced with pressures in a rapidly changing society with diverse, multi-cultural and ethnically rich families with a variety of needs and a disproportionate representation in child and adolescent mental health services. The globalisation of culture in a postmodern context and the power of Western orthodox practices contrasts with indigenous healing practices from the developing world. The chapter will consider the implications for employing a socially inclusive community model of practice in child and adolescent mental health services. The optimum methods and models of practice will be identified in order to achieve central government policy aims and measures of effectiveness against the multiple dimensions of culturally appropriate practice.

The need to develop child and adolescent mental health services (CAMHS) has attracted more attention in recent years due to increased demands on specialist resources by parents, teachers, social workers and primary health care staff. Attempting to meet the needs of children suffering emotional and behavioural problems as well as their carers/families has proved onerous. The evidence has suggested the need for policy and practice changes to ensure a sufficient range of provision and skills to improve the effectiveness and efficiency of CAMHS (Walker 2011).

A meta-analysis of comparative studies of adolescent stress found that the underlying causes of personal distress could be relatively similar between cultures (Bagley and Mallick 2000). Family dysfunction as perceived by the adolescent will, with other perceived stressors, therefore be a statistically significant predictor of various kinds of problem behaviours and emotional states in all ethnic groups. The conclusion is that there is possibly a measurable, culturally universal, aspect of the relations of adolescents to family and other stress in terms of emotional and behavioural problems, and impaired self-esteem. A causal pattern from stress to mental health problems cannot be demonstrated beyond reasonable doubt but it offers some evidence of important characteristics to consider.

There is a fine balance between normalising behaviour attributed to various causal factors and moving too quickly to subscribe to a formal psychiatric diagnosis or even formulating a hypothesis to be tested, inappropriately. Each way of conceptualising the presenting problem has implications for the short and long-term outcomes of assessment and intervention. A failure to recognise and acknowledge significant mental health problems could be just as damaging to the young person and others involved with them as could seeking to explain their behaviour with a definitive psychiatric diagnosis. In terms of cultural competence, this issue becomes crucial because different children will be affected in different ways by such a label.

For some refugee and asylum-seeking young people, for example, it could be a relief to have an explanation for feelings and behaviour that they find hard to make sense of, whereas for others it could exacerbate feelings of blame, guilt and self-loathing. The enduring social stigma of mental health problems, combined with institutionally racist practices, provides an overall context for these feelings to be repressed, displaced or acted out. Child abuse is now recognised as a problem of significant proportions in most cultures and the emotional and psychological consequences are well documented in the literature (Ferguson 2011). Yet despite compelling evidence practitioners still persist in ascribing other explanations for the behaviour or emotional state of minority ethnic individuals and families. Even within cultures there are marked differences based on gender. A recent study of Australian children, for example, who had been sexually abused found that boys were more likely to be in contact with public mental health services than girls. Abused boys and girls were more likely to receive a diagnosis of conduct disorder or personality disorder (Spataro et al., 2004).

Sociological perspectives

In addition to assessing the relevance of the orthodox developmental theories for a culturally competent understanding of child and adolescent development there are other, less prominent but as important resources for staff to draw upon to help inform therapeutic practice in this area. Sociology may be suffering from less emphasis in government policy and occupational standards guidance but it still offers a valuable conceptual tool to enable a rounded, holistic process of therapeutic assessment and intervention. Sociological explanations for child and adolescent mental health problems can be located in a macro understanding of the way childhood itself is considered and constructed by adults.

> Childhood is a social construction. It is neither a natural nor a universal feature of human groups but appears as a specific structural and cultural component of many societies.

> Childhood is a variable of social analysis. Comparative and cross-cultural analysis reveals a variety of childhoods rather than a single or universal phenomenon.

> Children's social relationships and cultures require study in their own right, independent of the perspective and concern of adults.

> Children are and must be seen as active in the construction and determination of their own lives, the lives of those around them and of the societies in which they live.

An examination of the experience of childhood around the world today shows how greatly varied it is, and how it has changed throughout history. Contemporary children in some countries are working from the ages of eight and are independent from the age of 14, whereas in other countries some do not leave home or begin work until they are 21 (Corsaro 2011). The conventional developmental norms show how adults construct childhood and therefore how to measure children's progress and detect mental health problems. They are, however, set down as solid absolutes and are based on notions of adults' fears about risk, lack of confidence in children, and rooted in adults' own childhood experiences. These theories have had positive effects but they have also restricted the field of vision required to fully engage with and understand children and adolescents from the diversity of cultures in a multi-ethnic society.

Identity formation

An ecological systemic theory of the psychosocial development of ethnic minority children and young people views development as a complex product of individual and contextual influences (Walker 2005). It is relatively easy to understand the impact of societal, media and government policy influences on the emerging self-awareness of ethnic minority children confronted by crude stereotypes. What is harder to appreciate is the subtle processes underway in younger children as they transit particular developmental stages while trying to develop a sense of individual identity based on the significance attached to group membership (Walker 2012). If we accept that the root of much psychopathology lies in disturbed or distorted developmental transitions then we must consider more carefully the additional burdens placed on ethnic minority children faced with more complexities to navigate.

The significance attached to particular ethnic group membership will itself of course be mediated by familial influences, genetic predisposition and temperament/personality characteristics unique to the individual. Thus in attempting to understand the experiences of children and young people we enter the paradox of trying to hold a singular concept of ethnic identity simultaneously with a multiple concept of individuation. Rather than accepting a systemic formulation of interactional influence or a linear psychodynamic formulation of personality development, we require a more sophisticated blend of the two.

Given that the developing child's earliest social relationship with the environment is with the primary caregiver, the quality of this relationship will determine to a large extent the child's subsequent approach to relating to the external world. As well as the inborn genetic and physical ability to organise experience, it will rely on the presence of others to provide certain experiences to develop adaptive capacities and strengths.

The developing child therefore builds mental representations from an early age made up of external experiences and the internal experiences of thoughts, imagining, memories and dreams. Accessible memory is thought to begin at around three years although what actually gets represented may not be historically accurate because experiences have to be interpreted. These mental representations contribute to the organisation of present behaviour when presented with new situations as well as acting as guidelines when we can identify situations which appear similar (Coulbeau et al., 2008). Previous experience therefore leads to the development of expectations of ourselves and others in certain settings where we tend to expect particular responses from others but also try to elicit them. This can explain the persistence of habitual ways of relating and the power of resistance to change which can be understood both as unconscious motivation as well as systemic circularity.

If we accept that the role of the primary caregiver is fundamental then it is reasonable to assume that their relationship with the external world based on their early experiences provides a chain of experiences linked to the earliest relationship between ethnic minority peoples and majority cultures. History demonstrates the distorted, prejudiced and discriminatory values enshrined in the treatment of ethnic minority people bought and sold as human cargo for slave traders on the back of scientifically flawed theories of race and human nature. The effects of these ideas and the values of white supremacy have tended to be understood in terms of economic and social disadvantage – the external symptoms that are more easily recognised, quantified and addressed. Indicators of poverty, unemployment and educational attainment can be used to illustrate the effects as well as provide a tangible focus for efforts to mitigate them.

However what is more difficult are the psychological effects of generational experiences of immigrant families subjected to overt hostility, discrimination and disregard. What are the accumulated internal interpretations of generations being treated as sub-human, worthless and a threat to 'normal' society? The responses and ways of adapting to life in a racist society are obviously as varied as the unique characteristics of individuals and families. However we can go some way to better understand the impact by accepting certain common experiences as possible options. These can provide us with clues about how to organise our work along more culturally competent lines.

The psychodynamic flight or fight response can serve as a useful starting point, offering as it does a framework within which to measure specific individual and family responses to stress or threat. We also need to keep in mind the notion of generational adaptation – a way in which each new generation of ethnic minority children and young people use the experiences of parents/ grandparents to screen or filter their own particular contemporary challenges. The evidence suggests a spectrum of adaptation to the psychosocial experience of discrimination from denial through to outright hostility. These have been captured and typified as the adopted black child found bleaching itself in the bath through to militant black power organisations seeking to influence younger generations of black children.

So in order to think more comprehensively about meeting the needs of children and young people from ethnic minority communities we need to start with the developing influences and interrelationships within their family. And we must understand these as fluid, organic processes rather than as static or unidimensional. In other words, within each separate family there will have been several periods of experiences and events that have shaped opinion and beliefs about themselves as a family and as a black family. For example a prevailing belief about white people may have been challenged or even overturned in the light of a new experience – negative or positive. Equally an assumption about the status of black people in society could have been reinforced and hardened over time.

So the focus for engaging troubled young people from ethnic minority families is in understanding the way individuals evolve and grow within a family environment. These are in turn influenced by the experience of being part of a community. In inner city areas where there is a richer cultural and ethnic mix of peoples there is a context for black families to test out their beliefs and assumptions with those who have a shared understanding. Neighbourhood interactions, informal or formal support systems and sources of information help families measure their individual experiences. As part of our work we need to be able to elicit these multiple levels of understanding in order to better assess the most effective culturally competent way to help.

Preventive practice

It is important not to be overly influenced by the negative connotations of causes, definitions and consequences. Too much emphasis on spotting emerging or established mental health problems in ethnic minority children and young people could unwittingly increase persecutory feelings and paranoia, thus provoking negative interactions that could lead to psychological disturbance. Focusing on pathology can distract from the critically important role of prevention. An ecological paradigm that understands the individual young person in an interactive relationship with their particular environment is a helpful point of departure in seeking to explain the internal and external stresses producing mental health problems. A health education framework that tackles the consequences of drug and alcohol misuse, combined with targeted early intervention and provision of accessible services in high-risk groups, is another important factor. Thirdly, given the significance in interpersonal problems as precipitating factors in the triggering of mental health difficulties, life skills education and training should be emphasised at known developmental crisis points such as pre-adolescence (Walker 2005).

The prevailing stigma associated with mental health problems is magnified in the context of minority ethnic children and young people as it gets mixed together with other notions reflecting the demonisation and denigration of young people. With black children there is an additional factor that sees their behaviour in terms of outside normality, primitive stereotypes and beyond control.

This is a powerful cocktail of ideas, and in the hands of a generally irresponsible media it can feed the general public with distorted or unrealistic perceptions of child mental health problems. Further stigmatisation can occur when mental health problems are linked with aggression, criminality and unpredictability. This can exaggerate public fears about young black people with mental health problems. Also people find it easier to see mental health problems belonging to others rather than themselves or their children. This protects against powerful feelings of vulnerability and that most threatening of ideas – that everyone is capable of becoming mentally unwell. We need to achieve a high level of personal insight as therapists if we are seeking to enter the troubled lives of clients and not be deflected or distracted by our own internal vulnerabilities.

Culturally competent practice is about understanding apparent psychological difficulties in a broader context than narrow diagnostic criteria or the absence/delay of developmental stages. It means working more in partnership with the child, young person and their family to understand their perspectives, in their language and in their belief systems. It is also helpful to consider why similar children and young people in similar circumstances have not succumbed to emotional or behavioural problems. What stopped them from having the same experience? What protective factors within the culture worked for them and might be replicated? Discovering this kind of evidence can enable you to formulate preventive strategies and reduce the risk/vulnerability factors for others in the community.

Establishing the therapeutic relationship

For staff working with children and young people the issue of engaging and establishing the therapeutic relationship becomes challenging when trying to incorporate culturally competent notions. You may worry about whether you need to start from scratch and learn a host of new concepts or you may feel that your existing methodologies and skills have stood the test of time and experience and require no change. As long as you accept that the issue is important enough to warrant examination of your existing practices then you have begun the process that will lead to a more culturally competent practice. The ability to engage with troubled children and adolescents is not easy at the best of times. At times of crisis or heightened anxiety from parents or other professionals it becomes particularly challenging. Paradoxically, by reflecting on cultural competence you may well find yourself managing these stressful events more easily. If we consider some of the potential barriers to engagement identified by, amongst others, Compton and Galaway (1999), we can begin to at least describe the elements likely to require particular attention.

Anticipating the other – this is connected to prejudging the situation and happens when we fail to listen carefully if we believe we know beforehand what the other person is going to say. This might be because of information provided by another source or our own stereotyped imagery about the situation being presented. The message and subsequent communication is anticipated and you drift into automatic language rather than reading between the lines of what the other person is saying.

Failure to make the purpose explicit – if you fail to make the purpose of contact explicit, then you and the client may have different, even contradictory ideas of what the purpose is and will interpret each other's communication in the light of different ideas. This may occur because of your anxiety about the likely reactions from the child or young person. As the subtle distortions continue, the two will be heading in entirely different directions.

Premature change activities – efforts to effect change will fail where you attempt to change without clearly understanding what the client wants and whether that change is feasible. Cultural competence requires that you make every effort to understand their point of view. To urge change prematurely may create a barrier to communication and can lead to directive approaches that are often ineffective in the absence of trust.

Inattentiveness – if your mind wanders during the contact, then the communication process is compromised. This happens when you are tired, thinking about the last or next client, bored or even frightened and upset. The situation you are confronted with might remind you about your own family or a deeply personal experience that has suddenly come into your mind and is distressing or distracting.

Client resistance – the barriers that some clients create can be thought of as forms of resistance against entering into a problem-solving process. They can stem from discomfort and anxiety involved in dealing with a strange person and a new situation, or from cultural or sub-cultural norms regarding involvement with service agencies and asking for help. Also some clients may be securing a degree of satisfaction from their problems.

In order to overcome these barriers to culturally competent engagement, you need to prepare fully and follow some relatively simple guidelines during the initial contact. These first steps to effective intervention can lay the future direction and pattern for the child or young person's contact with your agency and other helping relationships. Do not underestimate the importance of this. You need to examine your own inner prejudices and assumptions about the clients situation and try to suspend these to prevent them compromising good practice. Encountering early hostility, silence or non-compliance should be expected from reluctant or involuntary child and adolescent clients and not seen as reflecting your lack of skills.

Assessment as process

A wide definition of assessment will ensure your practice is empowering and culturally competent. It is important to think of assessment as a process rather than a one-off event. There should be a seamless transition from assessment to intervention in a circular process that includes the crucial elements of planning and reviewing. Once completed, the circle begins again at the assessment stage of the process and so on. Think of it as a continuous, perpetual movement, punctuated by a range of activities involving major or minor interventions in the lives of children and young people. Rather than adopting a *one-dimensional* view of assessment you could also perceive it as an intervention in itself – the very act of conducting an information-gathering interview could have a significant positive impact on a young person's wellbeing. The simple idea that someone cares and is prepared to listen to their story could be enormously comforting to a child or adolescent feeling lonely, isolated and with low self-esteem (Walker and Beckett 2011).

Accepting that assessment is an imperfect science is a good starting point for creative culturally competent practice. Also understanding that it is a dynamic process requiring high quality communication skills is very important. Dynamic in the sense that it is not static – information can become out of date, a family's functioning can deteriorate quickly, while the very act of assessment can affect that which you are assessing. Assessment is therefore a purposeful activity. It is the art of managing competing demands and negotiating the best possible outcome. It means steering between the pressures of organisational demands, legislative injunction, limited resources and personal agendas. It includes having the personal integrity to hold to your core values and ethical base while being buffeted by strong feelings.

An assessment should be part of a perceptual/analytic process that involves selecting, categorising, organising and synthesising data. If it is conducted as an exploratory study avoiding labels it can result in a careful deliberation of a young person's needs and not just fitting them into whatever provision exists. Remember that all assessments contain the potential for error or bias. These can be partly counteracted by following these guidelines (Coulshed and Orme 2012):

Improving self-awareness – so as to monitor when you are trying to normalise, be over-optimistic or rationalise data.

Getting supervision – which helps to release blocked feelings or confront denial of facts or coping with the occasional situation where you have been manipulated.

Being aware – of standing in awe of those who hold higher status or power and challenging their views when necessary.

Treating all assessments – as working hypotheses which ought to be substantiated with emerging knowledge, remembering that they are inherently speculations derived from material and subjective sources.

With government policy and organisational changes moving in the direction of more multidisciplinary team-working it is imperative that therapeutic assessment skills in the context of practice with other professionals are both authoritative and creative. The values and knowledge base of different staff from other agencies will be reflected in the way they think about and undertake assessment. Your contribution is crucial and depends on having the capacity to work with other colleagues in partnership. Working within a culturally competent framework will enable you to contribute important differences. Negotiation skills are paramount in order to enable you to challenge and confront when and where necessary to defend children and young people's therapeutic needs. Networking is considered a valuable attribute and you should be developing expertise in liaison, linking, communicating and convening meetings.

Multidisciplinary teams can become stressful places to work, particularly when the service is under pressure and energies are drained by resource shortages combined with high demand. It is easier to keep a low profile and grit your teeth in these circumstances rather than open up a painful or uncomfortable issue for discussion such as racism. However, you will gain respect by voicing concerns about the service or the clients and showing a willingness to tackle difficult issues. Being open, child-centred and demonstrating sensitivity to the team dynamics will be helpful to others who probably feel the same. Your broader understanding of children and young people in their cultural and socio-economic context together with your specific knowledge of psychotherapeutic processes will help clarify your distinctive and valued contribution.

Integrated intervention

An integrated culturally competent therapeutic model offers a concept of the mind, its mechanisms and a method of understanding why some children behave in seemingly repetitive, destructive ways. It offers the essential helping relationship involving advanced listening and communication skills with individuals or families. It provides a framework to address profound disturbances and inner conflicts within children and adolescents around issues of loss, attachment, anxiety and personal development in their authentic cultural context. Key ideas such as defence mechanisms, and the transference in the relationship between worker and client, can be extremely helpful in reviewing the work being undertaken, and in the process of supervision. The psychodynamic model in particular helps evaluate the strong feelings aroused in particular work situations, where, for example, a young person transfers feelings and attitudes onto the worker that derive from an earlier significant relationship. Counter-transference occurs when you try to live up to that expectation and behave, for example, like the client's parent (Walker and Thurston 2006).

It is a useful way of attempting to understand seemingly irrational behaviour based on Eurocentric assumptions and beliefs. The notion of defence mechanisms is a particularly helpful way of assessing male adolescents, for example, who may have difficulty expressing their emotions. The integrated model acknowledges the influence of past events/attachments and can create a healthy suspicion about surface behaviour while addressing the complexities in family interactions. The development of insight can be a particularly empowering experience to enable ethnic minority children and young people to understand themselves and take more control over their own lives.

A study found that parenting styles have an influence on whether young teenagers age 12 to 13 years engage in delinquent or antisocial activity (Smith et al., 2008). The study linked smoking and drinking to delinquency, and identified a substantial use of drugs in the age group. It also suggested that young people who had been victims of bullying, robbery or assault were more likely to commit offences. Researchers measured three personality dimensions: impulsivity, alienation, and self-esteem. Those who were victimised and those who offended tended to have lower self-esteem.

The study concluded that young people who witness parenting as arbitrary and inconsistent have a higher incidence of delinquency. Parents, however, who supervise children closely, but are happy to negotiate some degree of autonomy, are more likely to avoid teenage difficulties.

Families for whom parent education is unlikely to be a sufficient response to child management difficulties are those which feature maternal depression, socio-economic disadvantage and the social isolation of the mother. Extra-familial conflict combined with relationship problems also contribute to the problem severity and chronicity, and therefore affect the ability to introduce change. Parental misperception of the deviance of their children's behaviour is also a significant impediment to engaging in constructive family support (Walker 2013). In other words, simply referring any parent/carer to a parent education resource, or offering to convene a therapeutic group to parents/carers who cannot make use of the experience, is offering false hope. It can emphasise feelings of hopelessness and failure, reinforce guilt and undermine the relationship between client and practitioner.

Early intervention

The evidence demonstrates conclusively that one of the biggest risk factors in developing adult mental health problems is a history of untreated or inadequately supported childhood mental health problems (Green et al., 2005). Therefore it is imperative that counsellors and psychotherapists address this growing problem and offer their own distinctive contribution in the context of early intervention practice and various government health improvement programmes. Early intervention is often synonymous with preventive practice in child and adolescent mental health work (Walker 2012).

The principle of preparing people for potential difficulties is useful and resonates with proactive initiatives in schools, youth clubs and resources such as telephone helplines, Internet discussion groups and campaigns, to reach out to children and young people before they reach a crisis. But there is a dilemma in considering providing exclusive access to some of these resources for ethnic minority children. Whole school approaches to CAMH offer a socially-inclusive model and avoid the risk in further stigmatising some groups. Linking specific therapeutic interventions with agreed outcomes is problematic due to the network of variables potentially impacting on a child or young person's development. It is notoriously hard to accurately predict the effect of specific interventions, especially when there is a lack of a research and evaluation culture in an agency. Equally it is even harder to measure the impact of preventive or early intervention programmes because of the impossibility of proving that something did not happen.

Children and adolescents acquire different at-risk labels such as looked-after, excluded or young offender, affecting the variety of perceptions of their needs from the care system, education system or youth justice system. Ethnic minority children feature disproportionately in these categories. This can have a detrimental effect on efforts to build a coalition amongst different professional staff to intervene preventively. Each professional system has its own language and methodology with which to describe the same child, sometimes resulting in friction between agencies and misconceptions about how to work together and integrate interventions. Arguments over the *real* nature of a child's behaviour or the *correct* theoretical interpretation are a wasteful extravagance. In this climate, the mental health needs of such children can be neglected and the opportunity for thoughtful, preventive work missed.

As well as understanding why some children develop mental health problems, it is crucially important to learn more about those who in similar circumstances do not. Research is required to analyse the nature of these resilient children to understand whether coping strategies or skills can be transferred to other children. Positive factors such as reduced social isolation, good schooling and supportive adults outside the family appear to help. These are the very factors missing in socially excluded families who generally live in deprived conditions and suffer more socio-economic disadvantages than other children. Yet many of these children will not develop mental health problems.

One of the most important preventive approaches is helping children and young people cope with the stresses they face in modern society. Every generation has to negotiate the manifestations of stress in their wider culture therefore relying on ways used by former generations is not useful. This is challenging to practitioners who will naturally draw from their own experiences as an instinctive resource. However, the evidence suggests first in understanding the different *levels of stress* experienced by children and young people. Stress is a broad concept and includes a diverse range of experiences. The key is to ensure that the child themselves can categorise the level of stress according to their own cultural norms. For example, whether a bereavement is an acute or moderate stress, or whether parental separation/divorce is a severe and longer-lasting stress. What helps is enabling the child or adolescent to focus on what can be done to improve the situation rather than concentrating on negative feelings (Sempik et al., 2008).

Conclusion

Progressive ideas have been influencing practice in recent years as CAMHS staff seek ways of resolving the dilemmas inherent in modern practice that are constrained by managerialist values while demand for services increases. Cultural and socially inclusive practice is a useful paradigm that seeks to challenge received wisdom about what interventions are valid based on apparent empirical certainty. It articulates a theory that requires us to continually question the prevailing cultural orthodoxy and to deconstruct theories and practices based on old certainties. For staff aspiring to culturally competent practice, this is a valuable resource. Replacing conventional notions with a more flexible, less constrained perspective enables practice to embrace a plurality of intellectual resources from which to guide your work. The growth of the voluntary sector, devolved budgets, and decision making, horizontal management structures and contraction of local child and adolescent mental health services, are all stimulating the expansion of socially inclusive thinking as creative and innovative ways of delivering interventions (Walker, 2012).

Postmodern theorists have long argued the significance of power relationships within practice and argued for an analysis of how this impacts on intervention practice refracted through the prism of a commitment to social justice and human rights (Leonard, 1997). By attending more closely to the barriers constructed between yourself and clients you can begin to appreciate how professional language is a way of preventing cultural understanding rather than enabling useful communication. Narrative as a root metaphor can replace old modernist certainties derived from classic theoretical paradigms and medical models informing assessment and intervention practice. A more refined practice can become a dialogic-reflexive interaction between client and worker using language and the cultural construction of meaning to define the cultural parameters of the helping process.

If you are interested in a practice that seeks to challenge social inequalities and embrace radical ideas based on, for example, feminist or green politics, then you can begin with a structural analysis of power in society that produces exploitation of marginalised citizens. The postmodern paradigm advocates the importance of diversity, devolution, decentralisation and cultural interdependence. An integrated culturally competent model of practice drawing upon these notions searches for an understanding of the experience of the service user. Explanation or interpretation is still important, but in the context of social understanding that is pluralistic, where a range of cultural explanations can coexist and be part of a larger chain of enquiry that challenges discrimination in all its manifestations (Walker, 2012).

Therapeutic practices have become burdened by the managerial demands for efficiency, calculability, predictability and control. The relentless obsession with cost effectiveness implies that only things that can be counted are important, and that the standardisation controlled by technology ensures predictability. The ensuing conformity and globalisation of practice was foreseen by Dominelli many years ago (2008), who warned of the dangers of the privatisation of welfare services, new organisational structures in helping agencies and a redefinition of the therapeutic task that would lead to a deterioration in the relationship between worker and client, which professionals can testify to nowadays. This conflict between the bureaucratic context of your practice and the values that attracted you into helping work in the first place lie at the heart of cultural and socially inclusive practice. This offers a liberating perspective to help you locate your practice in the wider cultural context and within your personal value system.

References

Bagley, C. and Mallick, K. (2000). How adolescents perceive their emotional life, behaviour, and self-esteem in relation to family stressors: A six-culture study. In: *International Perspectives on Child and Adolescent Mental Health*. Oxford: Elsevier.

Compton, B. and Galaway, B (1999). *Social Work Processes* (6th ed.) Pacific Grove, CA: Brooks/Cole Publishing. Elsevier.

Corsaro, W.A. (2011) *The Sociology of Childhood*, New York: Sage.

Coulbeau, L., Royer, P., Brouziyne, M., Dosseville, F. and Molinaro, C. (2008). Development of children's mental representations: Effects of age, sex and school experience. *Perceptual Motor Skills*, 106 (1): 241–250.

Cousheld, V. and Orme, M. (2012). *Social Work Practice* 5th ed London: Palgrave Macmillan.

Dominelli, L. (2008). *Anti-Racist Social Work* London: Palgrave.

Ferguson, H. (2011). *Child Protection Practice* London: Palgrave Macmillan.

Green, H., McGinnity, A., Meltzer, H. et al. (2005). *Mental Health of Children and Young People in Britain 2004*. London: Palgrave.

Leonard, P. (1997). *Postmodern Welfare: Reconstructing an Emancipatory Project*. London: Sage.

Sempik, J. et al. (2008). Emotional and behavioural difficulties of children and young people at entry into care. *Clinical Child Psychology and Psychiatry*, 13 (2), 221–233.

Smith, P.K., Mahdavi, J., Carvalho, M., Fisher, S., Russell, S. and Tippett, N. (2008). Cyberbullying: Its nature and impact in secondary school pupils. *Journal of Child Psychology and Psychiatry*, 49 (4), 376–385.

Spataro, J., Mullen, P.E., Burgess, P.M. et al. (2004). Impact of child sexual abuse on mental health. Prospective study in males and females. *British Journal of Psychiatry*, 184, 416–421.

Walker, S. (2005). *Culturally Competent Therapy: Working with Children and Young People*, London: Palgrave.

Walker, S. and Thurston, C. (2006). *Safeguarding Children and Young People*, Lyme Regis: Russell House Publishers.

Walker, S. and Beckett, C. (2011). *Social Work Assessment and Intervention*. Lyme Regis: Russell House Publishers.

Walker, S. (2011). *The Social Workers Guide to Child and Adolescent Mental Health* London: Jessica Kingsley Publishers.

Walker, S. (2012). *Effective Social Work with Children, Young People and Families: Putting Systems Theory into Practice*, London: Sage.

Walker, S. (ed.) (2013). *Culture and Meaning in Child and Adolescent Mental Health in: Modern Mental Health* St. Albans: Critical Publishing.

8

BEING MIXED RACE[1]

Dinah Morley

I am one of many mixed race people who I feel are the forgotten ones. We don't look mixed race in a traditional sense. We look 'different' and people can't quite place where we are from, possibly Italian or South American. I now call myself mixed race and am happy with that because I don't care if other people mistake me for being white and expect me to say I'm white. What I do care about is that I don't fit in anywhere and that has given me issues of identity because if my skin was darker I could fit in with the mixed-race crowd and be accepted by the black crowd. But as it is I just look white and have to explain myself to people. (Mixed Experiences study, 2011)

It may be surprising to see a chapter on mixed-race children and young people in this book, but those working with children and young people of mixed race need to be aware of the particular risks to mental health/emotional wellbeing that may be present in the lives of those young people. This is not to pathologise the mixed-race child but rather to ensure that supports which are appropriate, relevant and robust are provided where they are needed. The comment above made by Carla, a young woman participant in the Mixed Experiences study (2011) with an Irish father and a Jamaican mother, shows how mixedness can create an 'outsider', even within the 'mixed race crowd'.

Proportionately, mixed-race children and young people under the age of 18 make up the fastest-growing group of young people in the United Kingdom – a trend borne out by the 2011 census data which indicated that there are now around 603,000 children of mixed race under the age of 18 in the UK population, compared with approximately 338,000 in 2001. On this basis alone, this population group is deserving of urgent consideration by practitioners in all services provided for children and young people, not least child and adolescent mental health services (CAMHS).

Children and young people of mixed race are not a homogenous group. They will have very different experiences of childhood depending on where they have grown up: what they look like, their skin colour and the way in which their family, school and community supports or undermines their mixedness. The group's extreme heterogeneity does not allow for a one-size-fits-all assessment of their needs and this is the challenge for practitioners.

Despite generally limited research, we know that mixed-race young people are likely to have had a significantly different experience in some aspects of growing up from their peers, both black and white. Some aspects of this experience can put them at greater risk of difficulties but can also promote resilience in quite distinct ways.

For example, a number of research studies have pointed to the racism these young people suffer at the hands of both black and white peers; the difficulties they experience in seeking a safe identity; the negative school experiences and the importance of family attitudes in ensuring that they become well-adjusted adults. All of these are often quite subtle and/or hidden experiences, and are set in the context of tensions they may face both within their families as well as within the wider communities in which they live.

While a wider reading of the statistical material suggests that people of mixed race are not necessarily over-represented in areas of social concern, there are some significant exceptions in some important domains. Owen and Statham (2009), looking at disproportionality in child welfare generally, note that children of mixed race are 'over-represented in every category – being high for children in need (5.0%) and more than double their population percentage (3.5%) amongst children on the child protection register (7.4%) and amongst those looked after, (7.8%)' (p. 22).

Data from the Costs, Outcomes and Satisfaction for Inpatient Child and Adolescent Psychiatric Services (COSICAPS) study (Tulloch et al., 2007) show that children of mixed race made up 7% of in-patients in the study that is, twice the percentage of all children. Numbers are small but significant, 26 children out of 403.

While mixed-race young people are doing less well overall in terms of GCSE passes, there is considerable variation within the mixed race category – with white/black Caribbean young people performing worst and at the same level as the black Caribbean group, which performs worst of all (Tickly 2004). These outcomes are closely linked to poverty, as measured by free school meal eligibility.

In 2013/14, young people from a mixed ethnic background accounted for 5% of young people in the justice system and while the total number of young prisoners has fallen over the past years, the proportion of mixed race prisoners is up by 42%. In the absence of further and more specific research this lack of proportionality must give cause for concern (Youth Justice Board, 2014).

Data are still hard to come by and, in so many publications – government publications included – black is still the default category for mixed race young people. In the popular discourse, and particularly around the period of the Obama elections, varying views have been expressed. People of mixed race largely want to be seen as who they are and for the mix that they are, but some do not and generally see themselves as black. Some again 'pass' as white and seem content with this. It is interesting that Obama is seen as the first black president of the United States.

This chapter draws on the in-depth research carried out in the field by Tizard and Phoenix (2002), Tickly et al. (ibid) and Aspinall and Song (2013). American studies that are based on populations whose experiences of racism and mixedness come from a very different background of history and legislation are not referenced here. The personal quotes from individuals are from the data collected through my small research project, Mixed Experiences, the findings of which are very similar to those of other small UK research projects into mixed race experiences, for example Alibhai Brown (2001), Katz (1996), Ali (2003), Ifekwunigwe (2004).

Identity and child focused issues

> Misidentification, to be considered not to be who one believes one is, to be denied preferred identities that are precious, are akin to psychological mutilation or annihilation. (2002 p. 44)

This quote from Bhui (2002) in his chapter on *Feeling for Racism* stresses the importance of the internal world in relation to racial discourse, of both black and white people. Bhui points to the potential attendant psychological damage inflicted by challenges to identity, which are felt keenly by most people of mixed race. This taking away of the identity of the child by, in most instances, adopting black as a default description for children of mixed race is tantamount to denying who they are and how they wish to be seen.

Identity is in any case a fluid concept throughout adolescence as young people strive to achieve their autonomy. It is exceptionally fluid for mixed-race young people who may want to be part of a 'group' and elect to be either white or black, and who may be very conflicted in making that decision. While Aspinall and Song (ibid), in their study of mixed race identities, show that these identities are fluid and perhaps not as important to some people of mixed race as might be supposed and can be assumed depending on circumstance and location. In inner-city environments it is easier to be mixed race.

The Mixed Experiences research, in common with other studies, showed how some young people of mixed race elected to be black as it seemed easier and gave them an instant group to belong to. In other cases, young people were seen as white and, while they lived their lives within this paradigm, they were uncomfortable doing so. Their white peers did not acknowledge their different ethnicity and this led to prejudiced/racist remarks being made which were deeply hurtful.

The situation is inevitably complex and will become more so as intermarriage becomes more commonplace. Aspinall and Song's study (ibid) demonstrates this and points to the fact that capturing this ethnic complexity does not happen currently.

> As the ethnic diversity of Britain has increased, driven by immigration dynamics and population mixing, leading to 'super-diversity', the census is no longer able to capture the new population, not least because – unlike the United States and Canada – Britain has no tradition in its censuses of asking an additional ancestry or ethnic original question.
>
> Such diversity has increased dramatically over the last few decades through population mixing, the emergence of new mixed/multiple identities and affiliations, and migration from an ever-increasing range of countries. (p22)

Skin colour is a significant factor in determining how mixed race people are seen and see themselves and can have a powerful influence on how friendship groups develop. Within the same family siblings can elect to be black, white or mixed depending on epidermal appearance. Whereas some young mixed-race people will identify strongly with one parent, possibly if only living with one parent, many struggle to give equal importance to the ethnicities of both parents, feeling disloyal if this cannot be achieved. For many, black is a safer place to be and even Barack Obama generally describes himself as black, thereby denying half of his ethnic inheritance. In his case he has never hidden the fact that his grandmother was white – visiting her prominently during his election campaign – but somehow it is easier for him to identify as black. This dilemma is described by Tina whose mother is Welsh and whose father is Guyanian.

> *My own experience has been that no white person will accept me as white, but if I claim blackness that is also denied. James Baldwin said that if people want to understand black people they have to become black. He was talking symbolically but I agree with him. Similarly, to understand the predicament of the mixed race person who is both the same and different requires an understanding (in the white person) of their own personal ambiguities and conflicts – those things in a person that are the same and different. This is hard work since it involves an alignment between self and 'other' and it's easier to view the mixed race person as 'other'.*

Family and being mixed race

It goes without saying that a secure and loving family is central to optimum growth and happiness of children and young people; however, it is important to reflect that, although parents may want to be supportive of their child's dual identity and to encourage their resilience, the parent of a mixed race child – unless they are mixed race themselves – can never fully understand the experience of their child. They can strive to list the benefits of mixedness but will never truly empathise with the deep sense of confusion that their child is feeling. The Mixed Experiences research (ibid) showed that often parents would try to be supportive but that they didn't connect with their child's feelings in a way that the child felt acceptable. Suhail, a young man with a Kenyan-Asian father and an English mother, describes the frustration he experienced as a result.

I was afraid to accept who I was, and being the oldest member of the family there was nobody else to talk to. I would get angry when my mum would try to explain that the world would view me differently to the way I viewed myself. I remember once smashing a plate in anger when my mother once brought up the subject.

In some instances, parents seem to have believed it was better to ignore the mixedness of their child as a way of helping her/him. As Emile points out, this is not done because parents don't care. However, he was left with no strategies to combat the racism he confronted, and which contributed to his hatred of one side of his racial inheritance.

I'm half Belgian, half Mauritian (my father is from the Island Mauritius). I'm very light skinned yet enough of my features have people ask me if I have African blood in me. My parents never really enlightened me about racial situations, not because they didn't care but probably because they wanted to 'protect' me. They probably thought that if you don't speak something it ceases to exist. Anyway, I got confronted with the whole race thing at a young age. I got called bastard child at school, heard my father being called names and things like that. At age 15 I had a confrontation with skinheads where I was beaten and threatened. I started to hate every drop of white blood I had in me.

In other cases families seem in total denial, or maybe just ignorant, of the likely difficulties their mixed race child could face. Thomas, who has an English mother and an absent Jamaican father, writes movingly of his frustration with his family and his admiration for his grandfather's change of view.

My grandmother would often try to calm me after some altercation at school by stating that I'm not really black, and my mother admitted that she remained oblivious to any difficulty I may face in life until walking with me as a toddler, when a passerby shouted the words 'nigger lover'. I don't think of anyone in my family as genuinely racist, but their cluelessness infuriated me then, as it does now. As a younger man, I had by far the most intelligent and insightful conversations with my grandfather: from a working class background (my grandmother's family repeatedly reminded her that she was marrying beneath herself), he had a bluntness which was far from charming but did me more favours. He bravely admitted to me that he was a racist before I was born, but that my arrival changed his perspective deeply.

Acceptance by the wider family has an impact, not only on the couple but on the children. Cyrus says that he and his (Asian) mother were accepted in the (English) father's family and it is interesting to see how class trumped race in his situation.

> *I was pretty sure they accepted me and accepted mum in a general sense but they weren't so concerned about skin colour. My dad always says that what his mum was interested in was what kind of class is she? They were obviously talking about what mattered in those days rather than race. On the other side my mum comes from a very small but strong community. They were very concerned about her marrying out.*

Class was a protector for a number of respondents to the Mixed Experiences study who described how their black 'professional' father validated the family's status.

There is often little contact with one side of a family because of geographical location. Young people may be able to maintain contact with distant families where there is enough money and a desire to visit as often as possible. In other cases language is a barrier. Where there is little possibility of contact children grow up with little knowledge of their full inheritance.

Tracey was keen to absorb both sides of her cultures but did not get very far, realising with incredulity that her white American father did not want her Chinese side properly acknowledged.

> *I asked my mother to teach me some Chinese. She speaks Cantonese only, but she taught me how to count from one to ten. Later I found out the reason she hadn't taught us while we were learning how to speak was because my father told her not to as he 'didn't want to feel like a foreigner in [his] own home.' This a source of frustration, annoyance, and a feeling of missing out for me and it also gives me a sense of rage, indignance at the arrogance and cultural superiority one can presume to have—toward his own wife, family! Why did they get married?*

The variety of experiences within families that are mixed is considerable. Unsurprisingly the young people who thrive are those whose families are supportive of their mixedness and encourage them to enjoy both sides of their inheritance. Where families cannot, or do not, acknowledge the negative experiences that their child might encounter the outcomes are less good.

School and the wider community

For many young people of mixed race the early primary school years are relatively free of any racism and rejection. From the Mixed Experiences research (ibid), it is evident that racist comments were directed to the mixed race children, but that they were not fully understood. This second comment from Cyrus points to the early damage these remarks can do.

> *I wasn't quite sure what they were talking about sometimes but they would suddenly talk about things and I was not quite sure what the hell they were going on about cos it was about monkeys and trees and things and that would really feel strange. But by and large I think I became more aware of the issues for myself really in my later teens.*

Secondary school experience was different. Young people, seeking autonomy, select themselves into groups of those who are like them and the person of mixed race has no group to join. This experience is evident from the findings of Ali (ibid) and Tizard and Phoenix (ibid) which show that other factors than race preoccupy children at the primary school age.

Kathleen confirms this aspect of her schooling:

> *Life was very simple until I was about 11 when I went to secondary school then it all changed! Secondary school was a nightmare! I was a bright kid and was eagerly looking forward to going 'big' school, but from the first day I was treated differently from the others, by both teachers and pupils. I was the only mixed race child in my school for the first four years... Some white teachers told me that they expected me to do better than the black kids because I had white blood in me, but the black kids hated me because of it. Other teachers told me I was doomed to failure because of my heritage.*

Tickly and colleagues (ibid), in their research in Birmingham schools, also note that mixed-race pupils experience racism not only from teachers but from both black and white pupils, something that is born out in much of the research across mixed-race issues. Teachers in the Birmingham sample explained the difficulties of their mixed race pupils as being because of identity issues and were convinced, incorrectly, that the majority of their mixed-race pupils lived in single white parent families, with mothers who could not deal with racist abuse. Tickly et al. demonstrate how this racism links with peer pressures to precipitate mixed race boys particularly into a downward spiral of poor achievement and 'unacceptable' behaviour.

A variety of tactics are deployed by mixed race young people to get through school days where these are experienced as being excluding and demoralising. These range from just getting their heads down and carrying on despite a hostile external environment, and escaping into music, drama, art and drugs. While these strategies are commonly seen in young people with other challenges in the adolescent years, for the mixed-race young person they are set against a backdrop of racism, confused loyalties and identity conflict. For some the process built their resilience and determination to succeed, others just wanted to get out as soon as possible. While these reactions are likely to be broadly similar for young people of any ethnicity and subject to the same experience of racism as any non-white child, the data show that for young people of mixed race, these responses have been strongly influenced by the attitudes of both pupils and teachers towards their mixedness. Some behaviours involved being the 'class clown' but in other cases protective behaviours were seen as disruptive and resulted in the young person being punished or moved to another class.

Other factors and racism

It has not been possible in this short chapter to look in depth at the full complexity of issues that potentially affect the mental health of mixed race children and young people. Geographical location, the sense of isolation even in the larger conurbations, access to the wider communities from which parents come, the stress engendered by mixed relationships and the absence of mixed-race role models all play a part in the heterogeneity of the mixed-race experience.

It will be evident from what has been presented here that there are specific challenges for children and young people of mixed race that can cause negative feelings about self to develop. Alongside this families struggle to support their mixed-race children appropriately and are not always able to help them develop their resilience in managing these challenges. While it is important not to pathologise mixedness, the disproportionality of mixed-race representation in key areas of social concern must be recognised and not ignored.

The Mixed Experiences research (ibid) identified the effect of racism, perpetrated by both black and white peers, as a key risk to mental health. This binary experience of racism was the most frequently reported damaging experience.

It is clear from a number of studies that, during childhood and adolescence, young people of mixed race experience real difficulties that, although apparently resolved for many, are likely to be imbedded in their minds. The qualitative data collected by various researchers (e.g. Katz (ibid), Alibhai-Brown (ibid), Morley (ibid)) identify difficulties in adulthood that are attributed, by the persons affected, to their mixedness.

Only further longitudinal research will allow us to fully understand these links, but we have enough evidence to alert us to the importance of recognising mixedness, in association with other factors, as a possible risk factor for mental health.

Despite, or possibly as a result of, considerable challenges, the Mixed Experiences study (ibid) found evidence of a developing resilience that enabled young people to reach a positive place as adults. Rosa, who described a difficult time in secondary school, now celebrates her Asian/Finnish experience.

I felt lucky that I wasn't 'boring' like everyone else. My name was always a talking point – I guess I do feel the same now. I always felt lucky to have seen three different ways of life, 2 religions, many different traditions etc. As much as I missed having one whole thing, I enjoyed being a part of so many different experiences.

Note

[1] **Mixed race**

In the British vernacular, the terms *race, culture* and *ethnicity* are frequently used interchangeably to describe the same phenomena in our 'multicultural society', referring to different countries of origin, shared religious practices and customs, epidermal difference and frequently class differences.

While accepting the fact that we are all one race and that genetically we differ very little from one another, between and across different groups, the term *mixed race* is used throughout as being the term most used and preferred by those who were consulted to inform the 2001 census (Aspinall et al., 2006). It is interchangeable to an extent with the terms *mixed heritage, multiple heritage, biracial, multiracial, mixed ethnicity* and *multi ethnic*.

References

Ali, S. (2003). *Mixed-race, Post-race: Gender, new ethnicities and cultural practices.* Oxford and New York: Berg.

Alibhai-Brown, Y. (2001). *Mixed Feelings: The complex lives of mixed-race Britons.* London: The Women's Press.

Aspinall, P., Song, M. and Hashem, F. (2006). *Mixed Race in Britain: A survey of the preferences of mixed race people for terminology and classifications.* University of Kent.

Aspinall, P. and Song, M. (2013). *Mixed Race Identities.* Basingstoke and New York: Palgrave Macmillan.

Bhui, K (2002). Feeling for Racism in Bhui, K. (ed.) (2002). *Racism and Mental Health.* London: Jessica Kingsley Publishers.

Ifekwunigwe, J. (ed.) (2004). *Mixed Race Studies: A reader.* London and New York: Routledge.

Katz, I. (1996). *The Construction of Racial Identity in Children of Mixed Parentage: Mixed Metaphors.* London: Jessica Kingsley Publishers.

Morley, D. (2011). *Mixed Experiences: A study of the childhood narratives of mixed race people related to risks to their mental health and capacity for developing resilience.* Unpublished thesis: City University.

Tickly, L., Caballero, C., Haynes, J. and Hill, J. in Association with Birmingham Local Education Authority (2004). *Understanding the Educational needs of Mixed Heritage Pupils.* London: Department for Education and Skills.

Tizard, B. and Phoenix, A. (2002). *Black, White or Mixed Race? Race and racism in the lives of young people of mixed parentage* 2nd. London and New York: Routledge.

Tulloch, S, Lelliott, P, Bannister, D, Andiappan, M, O'Herlihy, A, Beecham, J. and Ayton, A. (2007). *The Costs, Outcomes and Satisfaction for Inpatient Child and Adolescent Psychiatric Services (COSI-CAPS) study Report for the National Coordinating Centre for NHS Service Delivery and Organisation R&D (NCCSDO.)* London: HMSO.

Youth Justice Board (2014). *Youth Justice Statistics 2013/14 England and Wales.* London: Ministry of Justice.

9

THE ROLE OF SCHOOLS IN PROMOTING CHILDREN'S MENTAL HEALTH

Neil Humphrey

This chapter explores a range of issues relating to the role played by schools in promoting the mental health of children and young people. Attention is paid to universal provision of social-emotional learning as a means of preventing later difficulties, the school as a site for targeted/indicated work with children of or already experiencing problems and the potential utility of school-based universal mental health screening. Additional issues including strategic integration across schools and other services, training and development needs of school staff and the importance of effective implementation are also discussed.

What do we mean by mental health and why is it important?

What we mean and understand by 'mental health' and related terms (e.g. social and emotional wellbeing) is a critical starting point for this chapter. Mental health discourse is controversial, and there is a long-standing opposition to the traditional 'illness framework' in which it is viewed in terms of disease and disorder (Pilgrim, 2014; Rogers and Pilgrim, 2014). This is particularly the case when applied in the educational context (Graham, Phelps, Maddison and Fitzgerald, 2011), where it is seen by many as negative, stigmatising and problematising those experiencing difficulties (Link and Phelan, 2006). By contrast, the 'enhancement agenda' embodies a strengths-based approach to mental health that emphasises agency and resilience (Graham et al., 2011). Viewed through this lens, mental health is fundamentally about a state of wellbeing. This model has grown in popularity in recent years as wellbeing and 'the pursuit of happiness' (Centre Forum Commission, 2014) have come to the fore. Alongside this, the positive psychology movement has gained a significant foothold in education (Furlong, Gilman, and Huebner, 2014). However, some argue that in spite of its apparently positive focus, the enhancement agenda is still fundamentally about vulnerability and the diminishment of the human subject (Ecclestone and Hayes, 2008). One might also argue that an approach to understanding mental health that purposively ignores or underplays notions of distress risks drawing much-needed support away from those who need it most.

In this chapter, I take the middle ground between the two. The 'dual factor' approach views mental health as comprising two distinct dimensions, representing the experience of symptoms of psychological distress and adaptive functioning, respectively (Dowdy, Kamphaus, Twyford and Dever, 2014). Mental illness and health do not form a single continuum, but are instead seen as complementary but discrete continua (Dowdy et al., 2015). This model is illustrated in the National Institute for Health and Care Excellence's current definition, which posits emotional, social and psychological wellbeing as each including these distinct dimensions (e.g. emotional wellbeing is viewed in terms of happiness and confidence *and* anxiety and depression) (National Institute for Health and Care Excellence, 2013). This approach fits well with populist models of school-based provision (e.g. World Health Organization, 2004), in which universal interventions provide the basis for the promotion of adaptive functioning and resilience, and targeted approaches are implemented to remediate distress.

Experiencing positive mental health and wellbeing can be seen as part of every child's human rights (e.g. Article 6 of the Convention on the Rights of the Child notes the importance of being able to develop healthily – www.unicef.org/crc/) and is a fundamental component of a 'good childhood' (Dunn and Layard, 2009). Furthermore, longitudinal research demonstrates that the adaptive skills encapsulated in the enhancement view of mental health are important predictors of functioning in later life, including health and health-related outcomes (such as lower likelihood of obesity), and socio-economic and labour-market outcomes (such as higher income and being employed) (Goodman, Joshi, Nasim and Tyler, 2015). We also know that where significant distress is experienced (e.g. 1 in 10 children and young people experience clinically significant mental health problems – Green, McGinnity, Meltzer, Ford and Goodman, 2005), children are less likely to attend and achieve their potential in school (Colman et al., 2009) and more likely to be unemployed as adults (Farrington, Healey and Knapp, 2004). For these reasons, there has been a strong emphasis on early intervention and prevention (e.g. Allen, 2011).

Schools have the potential to play a central and highly effective role in promoting mental health. The nature of schooling provides a critical opportunity to effect positive change – it is universal, begins early in life and entails periods of prolonged engagement with children and young people (totalling around 15,000 hours – Rutter, Maughan, Mortimore, Ouston and Smith, 1979) during which effective identification and intervention strategies can be implemented. Schools play a central role in the lives of children and their families, and their reach is unparalleled (Greenberg, 2010). As a consequence, school-based mental health provision can influence outcomes for children who would not otherwise access the support they need through usual care pathways. As Greenberg notes, 'schools are the primary setting in which many initial concerns arise and can be effectively remediated' (2010, p. 28).

School-based mental health promotion in England: The policy context

In England, this potential has been recognised for some time, although efforts to tap into it have not always met with success. Under the Labour government (1997–2010), the seeds were sewn for more active and explicit consideration of child mental health and wellbeing through the installation of *Every Child Matters* (Department for Education and Skills, 2003). An influential review by Weare and Gray published in the same year (Weare and Gray, 2003) entitled *What works in promoting children's emotional and social competence and wellbeing?* brought to the fore the idea of universal social and emotional learning programmes in schools as a means to promote the skills that underpin positive mental health (Weare and Markham, 2005). The Department for Education and Skills subsequently commissioned the Behaviour and Attendance pilot via the National Strategies. Through this, the Social and Emotional Aspects of Learning (SEAL) programme was developed and was rolled out nationally in both primary (Department for Education and Skills, 2005) and secondary (Department for Children Schools and Families, 2007) schools. As the SEAL programme was primarily about universal provision (although some strands included materials intended for targeted delivery, such as the small group work component – Department for Education and Skills, 2006), this was followed up with the Targeted Mental Health in Schools (TaMHS) initiative (Department for Children Schools and Families, 2008), which was piloted from 2008 and launched nationally in 2010. Thus, under New Labour, the promotion of mental health and wellbeing was framed as a core component of education (indeed, wellbeing was included in the national school inspection framework used by the Office for Standards in Education, OFSTED). However, there were significant issues with this general approach. It was highly centralised and therefore left little room for autonomy and choice amongst schools. Initiatives were launched in quick succession, creating a sense of overload amongst schools (OFSTED, 2010). Both primary and secondary SEAL were brought to scale before their pilots had reported, meaning that problems experienced were not addressed ahead of their national launches (Humphrey, 2013).

Under the Coalition (2010–2015) and Conservative (2015 onwards) governments, the policy landscape pertaining to mental health promotion in schools has been mutable. In many ways, government policy post-2010 has arguably dismantled aspects of the education system that supported an emphasis on pupil health and wellbeing. In the early years of the Coalition, government endorsement of the SEAL programme was withdrawn, funding for participation in the National Healthy Schools programme was cancelled and the OFSTED inspection framework was changed to remove the explicit focus on personal development and wellbeing (although this has since been reinstated in the most recent revision – OFSTED, 2015). These policy shifts are part of a highly rationalist model of education, and reflect what Bonell et al. (2014) have termed the 'zero-sum game' view of attainment and health (e.g. academic attainment is singularly important in promoting economic competitiveness; any time spent on improving health and wellbeing in schools means less time for traditional academic instruction and thus produces lower attainment). However, this new landscape has also presented opportunities. The publication of new guidance on mental health promotion (Department for Education, 2014) provided an indication that it was indeed viewed as part of schools' remit and responsibilities. Since then, the government have launched MindEd (an online resource designed to help adults working with children and young people – including school staff – spot the early signs of mental health difficulties, www.minded.org.uk), and published their *Future in Mind* strategy document (Department of Health, 2015). As part of the latter, a pilot mental health training programme designed to raise awareness of mental health issues and promote effective joint working between schools and relevant external agencies (such as child and adolescent mental health service (CAMHS) teams) has been launched. Thus, there is increasing evidence of a shift back towards the view of schools and schooling as being central to effective mental health promotion for children and young people.

Schools as sites for universal prevention and promotion: The role of social and emotional learning

A prevalent feature in models of effective mental health provision (see, for example, World Health Organization, 2004) is the use of a tiered approach which begins with high-quality universal interventions designed to prevent the onset of difficulties through the development of supportive environments and the promotion of skills and competencies that help young people to thrive and engender resilience during difficult periods in their lives. While they are not the only possible sites for such provision (for example, such work can be community-based), for the reasons outlined earlier schools have become a primary context for delivery. One very popular approach to universal school-based provision is *social and emotional learning* (SEL). SEL programmes seek to help all children understand their emotions, manage their behaviour and work well with others. SEL theory suggests that developing such competencies in the context of a caring, participatory classroom environment engenders resilience to the onset of mental health difficulties because it fosters greater attachment to school, enables more effective coping in adverse circumstances and reduces risky behaviours (CASEL, 2007). Three recent meta-analyses have demonstrated that SEL interventions can make meaningful improvements to a range of outcomes for children, including their mental health (Durlak, Weissberg, Dymnicki, Taylor and Schellinger, 2011; Sklad, Diekstra, De Ritter, Ben and Gravesteijn, 2012; Wigelsworth et al., in press).

However, SEL programmes vary greatly in their design (e.g. component structure, prescriptiveness), and do not produce uniform effects. On the basis of the above analyses, there are certain features that appear to make a difference. First, more powerful effects are seen for programmes that embody the following 'SAFE' practices:

> *Sequenced* – the application of a planned set of activities to develop skills sequentially in a step-by-step approach

> *Active* – the use of active forms of learning such as role play

> *Focused* – the devotion of sufficient time exclusively to the development of social and emotional skills

> *Explicit* – the targeting of specific social and emotional skills (Durlak et al., 2011).

Additionally, interventions delivered by school staff (as opposed to external personnel) were shown to produce a more comprehensive range of positive outcomes (Durlak et al., 2011). Interestingly, though, no difference in effects between single component (e.g. curriculum only) and multi-component (e.g. curriculum and school ethos/climate) programmes was evident. Although this may seem counterintuitive, in all likelihood it is due to the fact that multi-component interventions are more complex and difficult to implement. Given the recent trend of importing established SEL interventions (see below), it is interesting to note that for many outcomes (including social and emotional competence, prosocial behaviour and emotional symptoms), these do not produce effects of the same magnitude as interventions being implemented in their country of origin (Wigelsworth et al., in press).

In England, the most well-known and widely implemented SEL initiative to date has been the aforementioned SEAL programme, which was being used in up to 90% primary schools and 70% of secondary schools by 2010 (Humphrey, Lendrum, and Wigelsworth, 2010). SEAL is described as, 'a comprehensive approach to promoting the social and emotional skills that underpin effective learning, positive behaviour, regular attendance, staff effectiveness and the emotional health and wellbeing of all who learn and work in schools' (Department for Children, Schools and Families, 2007, p. 4). The programme involves (a) the use of a whole-school approach to create a positive school climate and ethos, (b) direct teaching of social and emotional skills in whole-class contexts, (c) the use of teaching and learning approaches that support the learning of such skills, and (d) continuing professional development for school staff (Department for Children, Schools and Families, 2007). In both the primary and secondary school versions of SEAL, materials are presented thematically (e.g. 'New Beginnings', 'Getting On and Falling Out'). SEAL implementation in schools was supported by a number of guidance documents and materials pertaining to its different components (e.g. 'family SEAL', 'SEAL small group work'). Training was offered in local authorities (LAs) by behaviour and attendance consultants and other professionals working in children's services.

Evaluations of the SEAL programme produced very mixed results (see Humphrey, Lendrum and Wigelsworth, 2013, for a review) and attracted criticism on conceptual grounds (e.g. Craig, 2007; Ecclestone and Hayes, 2008). Following its discontinuation by the government in 2011,[1] there has been increasing proliferation of universal SEL programmes imported from other countries, with an emphasis on those that are deemed to be 'evidence-based'. Given the lack of centralisation in education policy in this area post-2010, this has often been driven by researchers and third sector organisations. For example, an adapted version of the Promoting Alternative Thinking Strategies (PATHS) curriculum, originally developed in the United States (Kusche and Greenberg, 1994) and well validated by research (see Allen, 2011), is currently being implemented in a large number of schools in locations across the United Kingdom (including Manchester, Birmingham, London, Glasgow, Swansea and Belfast). However, three recent trials of this intervention (Humphrey et al., 2015; Little et al., 2012; Ross, Sheard, Cheung, Elliott and Slavin, 2011) have produced very mixed findings, perhaps reinforcing the need to ensure that due consideration is given to context and cultural adaptation of programmes developed elsewhere in the world.

Schools as sites for targeted/indicated mental health interventions

Research into targeted/indicated provision reveals that school-based interventions can be beneficial for children and young people who are at risk of or already experiencing mental health difficulties (e.g. Gansle, 2005; Horowitz and Garber, 2006; Shucksmith, 2007; Wilson and Lipsey, 2007). As with universal approaches, systematic reviews and meta-analyses (ibid) reveal useful information about what does and does not appear to make a difference in their efficacy. So, for example, Wilson and Lipsey's (2007) meta-analysis of interventions to address externalising difficulties found that treatment modality had little bearing on the size of effects produced by different interventions, although this is perhaps because of the predominance of cognitive-behavioural approaches in the research literature (Shucksmith, 2007). In line with the findings of Durlak et al. (2011) for universal SEL, there is also limited evidence to suggest that multi-component approaches are any more effective than less complex interventions (Shucksmith, 2007). In terms of frequency, length and duration, once or twice weekly sessions are common amongst efficacious interventions, which tend to be of much longer duration for externalising difficulties than for internalising symptoms, perhaps because the former are seen as more deep-rooted and intense (Shucksmith, 2007).

Given that targeted/indicated interventions might traditionally be considered the remit of health professionals (e.g. those working in CAMHS), an interesting question that arises is whether teachers and other school staff can be equally effective intervention agents when such work is based in school, rather than clinical contexts. Notwithstanding the issues this question provokes in relation to the role and responsibilities of the modern teacher, the evidence base unfortunately does not permit a clear answer, as almost all studies report delivery being undertaken by external specialists rather than school staff (Shucksmith, 2007). This is an important avenue for future research, especially given the major cuts to child mental health services in two-thirds of LAs since 2010 (YoungMinds, 2013), which have had the effect of increasing pressure on schools to 'pick up the pieces'

(O'Hara, 2014). Thus, targeted/indicated mental health interventions that are located in and led by schools may increase if current levels of unmet need are to reduce.

In England, the most well-known and widely implemented school mental health initiative to date that has involved targeted work is known as Targeted Mental Health in Schools (TaMHS) (Department for Children Schools and Families, 2008). TaMHS was launched towards the end of the New Labour period – initially as a large pathfinder pilot and subsequently as a national scale-up – and was designed to build on and complement the universal platform provided by SEAL (see earlier). TaMHS was not a single intervention but rather a framework provided to schools through which they were able to develop locally crafted models of targeted support for children with nascent or established mental health difficulties. TaMHS was based on two key tenets: (i) that intervention selection be informed by the evidence base for school mental health provision and (ii) that the initiative should support strategic integration across agencies involved in the delivery of CAMHS. Beyond these principles, TaMHS was very much about local tailoring of support to context and need. Supported by a range of external agents and support systems, schools undertook activities and interventions in three key areas: (i) child-focused support (e.g. targeted/indicated interventions, supplemented by universal provision, (ii) parent-focused support (e.g. training to improve parenting skills and confidence) and (iii) staff-focused support (e.g. staff training on mental health-related issues) (Deighton et al., 2013). A randomised trial conducted as part of the national evaluation of TaMHS demonstrated that it led to significant and meaningful reductions in externalising difficulties amongst at-risk children in primary schools, but there was no evidence of a similar effect on internalising symptoms. Secondary school data produced completely null results. The evaluation also demonstrated that TaMHS led to significant increases in school provision of a range of interventions and improved collaboration between schools and specialist mental health services, but these actions were not themselves associated with the improvements in outcomes observed (Wolpert et al., 2015). Thus, while there was evidence that TaMHS was effective in improving some outcomes for certain children, the mechanisms underpinning this remain unclear.

Schools as sites for early identification of mental health difficulties

It has been argued that truly effective and comprehensive mental health provision in schools requires us to adopt a population-based approach to identification of children experiencing difficulties. Universal screening, in which all pupils in a school undergo periodic, brief assessments designed to identify those most at-risk (who may then be referred for more detailed assessment and/or intervention), has been the subject of recent calls for action (see, for example, Williams, 2013). Dvorsky et al. (2014) claim three key benefits of such a system. First, universal screening means that all children and young people are assessed. This should have the effect of reducing the number of those being overlooked compared to the existing 'refer-test-place' and 'wait to fail' models that are currently used (Dowdy, Ritchey and Kamphaus, 2010; Glover and Albers, 2007). Second, universal screening offers a more systematic, data-driven approach to mental health provision in schools. Third, universal screening can offer significant cost-savings as it should lead to earlier intervention, which is less intensive and expensive than indicated interventions for more severe or entrenched problems.

Despite these apparent benefits, universal mental health screening is extremely rare. For example, only 2% of schools in the United States use this approach as part of their routine practice (Romer and McIntosh, 2005). This contrasts sharply with screening for physical health indicators (e.g. vision, hearing), which have been universally assessed for decades (Dowdy et al., 2010; Williams, 2013). What accounts for this discrepancy? It may reflect the fact that mental health has traditionally not been given equal weight to physical health in public policy (H. M. Government, 2010). The stigma associated with mental health is also a likely contributory factor (Dowdy et al., 2010; Evans-Lacko et al., 2014). In considering the potential of universal screening as a component of a comprehensive approach to school-based mental health provision, there are numerous questions to be addressed, including those of social validity (e.g. is screening acceptable, feasible and perceived as useful by stakeholders such as teachers?), definition and conceptualisation (see earlier section – what we mean by mental health influences what and how we screen), design and implementation (e.g. measure selection, linking to referral and intervention systems), psychometric considerations (e.g. are available instruments reliable and valid?), diversity (e.g. taking into account cultural variation) and costs and benefits (e.g. are the human, financial and material costs of universal screening justified by the improvements in provision and outcomes they bring?).

The importance of high-quality implementation in school mental health

In order to produce successful outcomes for children and young people, the various dimensions of school mental health provision discussed thus far all depend heavily on effective implementation. Implementation can be defined as the putting into practice of an intervention (Humphrey, 2013). Many years of study have shown that interventions are rarely implemented as designed, and that variability in implementation is associated with variability in outcomes. Put simply, implementation matters (Durlak and DuPre, 2008). The various dimensions of implementation include *fidelity* (e.g. was the intervention delivered as intended by its developers?), *dosage* (e.g. how much of the intervention was delivered?), *adaptation* (e.g. what changes/modifications were made and why?), *quality* (e.g. how well was the intervention delivered?), *participant responsiveness* (e.g. did recipients engage with the intervention?), *reach* (e.g. was the intervention delivered to all intended recipients?) and *programme differentiation* (e.g. to what extent was the intervention distinct from usual practice?). By way of an example, the evaluation of the Kidsmatter school mental health initiative in Australia (which, like the aforementioned TaMHS, utilised a framework approach) demonstrated that quality of implementation was a key moderator of both social-emotional and academic outcomes (Askell-Williams, Dix, Lawson and Slee, 2013; Dix, Slee, Lawson and Keeves, 2012).

Given their importance, attention should be paid to the factors known to affect these dimensions. If we know what these factors are, we can build a model for the optimal conditions for effective implementation that can be communicated to schools as part of the programme dissemination process. Drawing on reviews by Durlak and DuPre (2008), Forman, Olin, Hoagwood and Crowe (2009) and Greenberg et al. (2005), these factors can be thought of in terms of *preplanning and foundations* (e.g. is there a need, readiness and capacity for change in a given school?), the *implementation support system* (e.g. is training and/or external support available?), the *implementation environment* (e.g. does the school leader provide appropriate support for the intervention? Are the necessary resources available?), *implementer factors* (e.g. do staff have both the will and skill to implement a given intervention effectively?), and *programme characteristics* (e.g. is the intervention developmentally appropriate?). By extension, consideration also needs to be given to more macro-level influences including government policies, leadership and human capital (Domitrovich, 2008).

Mental health training and development needs of school staff

As the role of schools in promoting positive mental health and preventing the onset or escalation of difficulties increases, it is critical to consider the training and development needs of staff. Recent initiatives (see earlier section) notwithstanding, it is fair to say that this is an area that has been largely neglected. For example, in a recent scoping survey of school mental health provision in England, two-thirds of primary schools and one-half of secondary schools reported that the individual(s) with primary responsibility for pupils' mental health support had no specialist training. Furthermore, few schools considered training and supervision of staff as a key part of their overall approach to mental health promotion (Vostanis, Humphrey, Fitzgerald, Wolpert and Deighton, 2013). These findings are in sharp contrast to literature which suggests teachers and other school staff express concern about the lack of training they have received (see for example Kidger, Gunnell, Biddle, Campbell and Donovan, 2010; Rothì, Leavey and Best, 2008).

Although the recent initiatives noted earlier in this chapter (e.g. MindEd, Future in Mind) provide clear steps in the right direction regarding staff training and development, many have argued that this is insufficient given the increasing centrality of schools in the child and adolescent mental health system. Thus, calls have been aired for mental health to be a fundamental aspect of initial teacher training with subsequent mandated professional development on an ongoing basis (House of Commons Health Committe, 2014). Clarity is required, however, regarding the content of such training. A comprehensive training and development model inclusive of issues pertaining to core concepts (e.g. definitions, prevalence), identification, assessment, referral, intervention, evaluation and monitoring, and interagency working is clearly preferable, but this needs to be balanced against the capacity of an already pressurised initial teacher education system and (arguably) limited space for continuing professional development amongst serving teachers in England (currently only five days per school year).

The research base on teacher training around mental health issues is rather limited (Loades and Mastroyannopoulou, 2010), but that which has been published is promising. For example, Jorm, Kitchener, Sawyer, Scales and Cvetkovski (2010) reported on the trialling of a 'Youth Mental Health First Aid' course for teachers, which was found to improve teachers' knowledge and understanding, reduce some aspects of mental health stigma and increase their confidence in providing help to pupils. The training also yielded an indirect effect on pupils, who reported receiving more information about mental health from school staff. Most of these changes were sustained at six-month follow-up. Although the authors found no effects on the levels of support provided by teachers or indeed the mental health of their students, this perhaps reflects a lack of capacity in schools, and thus reinforces the need for change at all levels of the system (that is, no amount of training and professional development is likely to impact upon pupils' mental health unless appropriate provision is in place for referral and intervention).

Effective interagency working in school mental health

School mental health provision does not operate in a vacuum, and school staff are thus most appropriately viewed as part of a multi-professional team who work together in the best interests of children and young people. In the traditional CAMHS strategic framework, they are located in the first tier of support, alongside other professionals working in universal services (e.g. general practitioners), although of course the nature of service delivery necessitates collaboration with specialist staff (e.g. psychologists, social workers) working in the upper tiers. Mental health can be seen as a microcosm of the wider challenges associated with multi-agency collaboration in children's services more generally. Over a decade ago, research by Pettit (2003) highlighted key issues relating to effective joint working between schools and CAMHS that included the influence of different organisational and professional cultures, expectation management, communication and sharing of information. The introduction of a standardised procedure for gathering, recording and sharing of information (the Common Assessment Framework) alongside initiatives designed to promote its use as part of a broader pattern of improved collaboration between schools and specialist mental health services (such as the aforementioned TaMHS) made some headway in this regard, but recent research suggests that there are still considerable challenges to be addressed (Fazel, Hoagwood, Stephan and Ford, 2014). Given this, the provision of effective joint working as a central part of the pilot mental health training developed following the publication of Future in Mind is most welcome.

Conclusion

In this chapter, I have explored a range of issues relating to the role played by schools in promoting the mental health of children and young people. Working from a dual-factor model, I have argued that schools have the potential to play a central and highly effective role as a hub for early identification, promotion of positive mental health and remediation of difficulties. Accordingly, three key areas of activity have been discussed – universal prevention and promotion, targeted/indicated interventions and universal screening. Moderators of the success (or failure) of these activities have also been presented, including strategic integration across schools and other services, training and development needs of school staff and the importance of effective implementation.

Note

[1] Despite being no longer endorsed by the government, SEAL is still implemented in many schools (www.sealcommunity.org/).

References

Allen, G. (2011). *Early intervention: the next steps*. London: HM Government.

Askell-Williams, H., Dix, K.L., Lawson, M.J. and Slee, P. T. (2013). Quality of implementation of a school mental health initiative and changes over time in students' social and emotional competencies. *School Effectiveness and School Improvement*, 24, 357–381.

Bonell, C., Humphrey, N., Fletcher, A., Moore, L., Anderson, R. and Campbell, R. (2014). Why schools should promote students' health and wellbeing. *BMJ (Clinical Research Ed.)*, 348, g3078.

CASEL. (2007). *How evidence-based SEL programs work to produce greater student success in school and life*. Chicago: CASEL.

Centre Forum Commission. (2014). *The pursuit of happiness: a new ambition for our mental health*. London: Centre Forum Commission.

Colman, I., Murray, J., Abbott, R., Maughan, B., Kuh, D., Croudace, T. J. and Jones, P.B. (2009). Outcomes of conduct problems in adolescence: 40 year follow-up of national cohort. *British Medical Journal*, 338, a2981–a2981.

Craig, C. (2007). *The potential dangers of a systematic, explicit approach to teaching social and emotional skills (SEAL)*. Glasgow: Centre for Confidence and Wellbeing.

Deighton, J., Humphrey, N., Wolpert, M., Patalay, P., Belsky, J. and Vostanis, P. (2015). An evaluation of the implementation and impact of England's mandated school-based mental health initiative in elementary schools. *School Psychology Review*, 44, 117–139.

Deighton, J., Patalay, P., Belsky, J., Humphrey, N., Vostanis, P., Fugard, A., … Wolpert, M. (2013). Targeted mental health provision in primary schools for children with behavioural difficulties: results of a national randomized controlled trial. *Psychology of Education Review*, 37, 40–47.

Department for Children Schools and Families (2007). *Social and emotional aspects of learning (SEAL) programme: guidance for secondary schools*. Nottingham: DCSF Publications.

Department for Children Schools and Families (2008). *Targeted Mental Health in Schools Project*. Nottingham: DCSF Publications.

Department for Education (2014). *Mental health and behaviour in schools*. London: DFE Publications.

Department for Education and Skills (2003). *Every child matters*. Nottingham: DfES Publications.

Department for Education and Skills (2005). *Primary social and emotional aspects of learning (SEAL): guidance for schools*. Nottingham: DES Publications.

Department for Education and Skills (2006). *Excellence and enjoyment: social and emotional aspects of learning (Key Stage 2 small group activities)*. Nottingham: DfES Publications.

Department of Health. (2015). *Future in mind: promoting, protecting and improving our children and young people's mental health and wellbeing*. London: Department of Health.

Dix, K.L., Slee, P.T., Lawson, M.J. and Keeves, J.P. (2012). Implementation quality of whole-school mental health promotion and students' academic performance. *Child and Adolescent Mental Health*, 17, 45–51.

Domitrovich, C. (2008). Maximizing the implementation quality of evidence-based preventive interventions in schools: A conceptual framework. *Advances in School Mental Helarth Promotion*, 1, 6–28.

Dowdy, E., Furlong, M., Raines, T.C., Bovery, B., Kauffman, B., Kamphaus, R.W., ... Murdock, J. (2015). Enhancing school-based mental health services with a preventive and promotive approach to universal screening for complete mental health. *Journal of Educational and Psychological Consultation*, 25, 178–197.

Dowdy, E., Kamphaus, R.W., Twyford, J.M. and Dever, B.V. (2014). Culturally competent behavioral and emotional screening. In M. D. Weist (ed), *Handbook of school mental health* (pp. 311–321). New York, NY: Springer.

Dowdy, E., Ritchey, K. and Kamphaus, R.W. (2010). School-Based screening: A population-based approach to inform and monitor children's mental health needs. *School Mental Health*, 2, 1–11.

Dunn, J. and Layard, R. (2009). *A Good Childhood: Searching for Values in a Competitive Age*. London: Penguin.

Durlak, J.A, Weissberg, R.P., Dymnicki, A.B., Taylor, R.D. and Schellinger, K.B. (2011). The impact of enhancing students' social and emotional learning: a meta-analysis of school-based universal interventions. *Child Development*, 82, 405–32.

Durlak, J.A. and DuPre, E.P. (2008). Implementation matters: a review of research on the influence of implementation on program outcomes and the factors affecting implementation. *American Journal of Community Psychology*, 41, 327–50.

Ecclestone, K. and Hayes, D. (2008). *The Dangerous Rise of Therapeutic Education*. London: Routledge.

Evans-Lacko, S., Courtin, E., Fiorillo, A., Knapp, M., Luciano, M., Park, A.L., ... Thornicroft, G. (2014). The state of the art in European research on reducing social exclusion and stigma related to mental health: A systematic mapping of the literature. *European Psychiatry*, 29, 381–389.

Farrington, D.P., Healey, A. and Knapp, M. (2004). Adult labour market implications of antisocial behaviour in childhood and adolescence: findings from a UK longitudinal study. *Applied Economics*, 36, 93–105.

Fazel, M., Hoagwood, K., Stephan, S. and Ford, T. (2014). Mental health interventions in schools in high-income countries. *The Lancet Psychiatry*, 377–387.

Forman, S., Olin, S., Hoagwood, K. and Crowe, M. (2009). Evidence-based interventions in schools: Developers' views of implementation barriers and facilitators. *School Mental Health*, 1, 26–36.

Furlong, M.J., Gilman, R. and Huebner, E.S. (2014). *Handbook of positive psychology in schools* (2nd ed.). London: Routledge.

Gansle, K. A. (2005). The effectiveness of school-based anger interventions and programs: A meta-analysis. *Journal of School Psychology*, 43, 321–341.

Glover, T.A. and Albers, C.A. (2007). Considerations for evaluating universal screening assessments. *Journal of School Psychology*, 45, 117–135.

Goodman, A., Joshi, H., Nasim, B. and Tyler, C. (2015). *Social and emotional skills in childhood and their long-term effects on adult life.* London: Early Intervention Foundation.

Graham, A., Phelps, R., Maddison, C. and Fitzgerald, R. (2011). Supporting children's mental health in schools: Teacher views. *Teachers and Teaching: Theory and Practice*, 17, 479–496.

Green, H., McGinnity, A., Meltzer, H., Ford, T. and Goodman, R. (2005). *Mental health of children and young people in Great Britain.* Newport: Office for National Statistics.

Greenberg, M., Domitrovich, C., Graczyk, P., Zins, J. and Services, C. for M. H. (2005). *The study of implementation in school-based preventive interventions: Theory, research, and practise.* Rockville: CMHS.

Greenberg, M.T. (2010). School-based prevention: Current status and future challenges. *Effective Education*, 2, 27–52.

H. M. Government. (2010). *Healthy lives, healthy people: Our strategy for public health in England.* London: HM Government.

Horowitz, J.L. and Garber, J. (2006). The prevention of depressive symptoms in children and adolescents: A meta-analytic review. *Journal of Consulting and Clinical Psychology*, 74, 401–15.

House of Commons Health Committe. (2014). *Children's and adolescent's mental health and CAMHS: Third report of session 2014-15.* London: House of Commons.

Humphrey, N. (2013). *Social and Emotional Learning: A Critical Appraisal.* London: Sage Publications.

Humphrey, N., Barlow, A., Wigelsworth, M., Lendrum, A., Pert, K., Joyce, C., ... Turner, A. (2015). *Promoting Alternative Thinking Strategies (PATHS): Evaluation report.* London: Education Endowment Foundation.

Humphrey, N., Lendrum, A. and Wigelsworth, M. (2010). *Secondary social and emotional aspects of learning (SEAL): national evaluation.* Nottingham: Department for Education.

Jorm, A.F., Kitchener, B.A., Sawyer, M.G., Scales, H. and Cvetkovski, S. (2010). Mental health first aid training for high school teachers: A cluster randomized trial. *BMC Psychiatry*, 10, 51.

Kidger, J., Gunnell, D., Biddle, L., Campbell, R. and Donovan, J. (2010). Part and parcel of teaching? Secondary school staff's views on supporting student emotional health and well-being. *British Educational Research Journal*, 36, 919–935.

Kusche, C. and Greenberg, M.T. (1994). *The PATHS curriculum*. Seattle, WA: Developmental Research and Programs.

Link, B.G. and Phelan, J.C. (2006). Stigma and its public health implications. *The Lancet*, 367, 528–529.

Little, M., Berry, V., Morpeth, L., Blower, S., Axford, N., Taylor, R., ... Tobin, K. (2012). The Impact of three evidence-based programmes delivered in public systems in Birmingham, UK. *Journal of Children's Services*, 6, 338–350.

Loades, M.E. and Mastroyannopoulou, K. (2010). Teachers' recognition of children's mental health problems. *Child and Adolescent Mental Health*, 15, 150–156.

National Institute for Health and Care Excellence. (2013). *Social and emotional wellbeing for children and young people*. London.

O'Hara, M. (2014). Teachers left to pick up pieces from cuts to youth mental health services. *The Guardian, April 25*, accessed at: www.theguardian. com/education/2014/apr/15/pupils-mental-health-cuts-services-stress-teachers.

OFSTED. (2010). *The National Strategies: a review of impact*. London: OFSTED.

OFSTED. (2015). *The common inspection framework: education, skills and early years*. London: OFSTED.

Pettit, B. (2003). *Effective joint working between Child and Adolescent Mental Health Services (CAMHS) and schools*. Nottingham: DfES Publications.

Pilgrim, D. (2014). *Key concepts in mental health*. London: Sage Publications.

Rogers, A. and Pilgrim, D. (2014). *A sociology of mental health and illness*. Buckingham: Open University Press.

Romer, D. and McIntosh, M. (2005). The roles and perspectives of school mental health professionals in promoting adolescent mental health. In D.L. Evans, E.B. Foa, R.E. Gur, H. Hendin, C.P. O'Brien, M. Seligman and B.T. Walsh (eds), *Treating and preventing adolescent mental health disorders* (pp. 598–615). Oxford: Oxford University Press.

Ross, S.M., Sheard, M.K., Cheung, A., Elliott, L. and Slavin, R. (2011). Promoting primary pupils' social-emotional learning and pro-social behaviour: longitudinal evaluation of the Together 4 All Programme in Northern Ireland. *Effective Education*, 3, 61–81.

Rothì, D.M., Leavey, G. and Best, R. (2008). On the front-line: Teachers as active observers of pupils' mental health. *Teaching and Teacher Education*, 24, 1217–1231.

Rutter, M., Maughan, B., Mortimore, P., Ouston, J. and Smith, A. (1979). *Fifteen thousand hours: secondary schools and their effects on children*. Cambridge, MA: Harvard University Press.

Shucksmith, J. (2007). *Mental wellbeing of children in primary education (targeted / indicated activities)*. Teeside: University of Teeside.

Sklad, M., Diekstra, R., De Ritter, M., Ben, J. and Gravesteijn, C. (2012). Effectiveness of school-based universal social, emotional, and behavioral programs: Do they enhance students' development in the area of skills, behavior and adjustment? *Psychology in the Schools*, 49, 892–909.

Vostanis, P., Humphrey, N., Fitzgerald, N., Wolpert, M. and Deighton, J. (2013). How do schools promote emotional wellbeing among their pupils? Findings from a national scoping survey of mental health provision in English schools. *Child and Adolescent Mental Health*, 18, 151–157.

Weare, K. and Gray, G. (2003). *What works in promoting children's emotional and social competence and wellbeing?* Nottingham: DfES Publications.

Weare, K. and Markham, W. (2005). What do we know about promoting mental health through schools? *Promotion and Education*, 12, 4–8.

World Health Organization. (2004). *Mental health programmes in schools*. Geneva: WHO.

Wigelsworth, M., Lendrum, A., Oldfield, J., Scott, A., Ten-Bokkel, I., Tate, K. and Emery, C. (in press). The influence of trial stage, developer involvement and international transferability on the outcomes of universal social and emotional learning outcomes: A meta-analysis. *Cambridge Journal of Education*.

Williams, S. (2013). Bring in universal mental health checks in schools. *British Medical Journal*, 5478, 24–26.

Wilson, S.J. and Lipsey, M.W. (2007). School-based interventions for aggressive and disruptive behavior: update of a meta-analysis. *American Journal of Preventive Medicine*, 33(2 Suppl), S130–43.

YoungMinds. (2013). *Local authorities and CAMHS budgets 2012/2013*. London: YoungMinds.

10

FROM OUTREACH TO REACHING OUT: A RELATIONAL APPROACH TO MENTAL HEALTH WITHIN THE COMMUNITY

Nick Barnes

Introduction: Setting the scene

Over recent years, there has been a heightened awareness of a 'national crisis' regarding care and support for children and young people's mental health and emotional wellbeing (Cooper, 2014). There has been a realisation of growing levels of need that are significant and profound (Collishaw et al., 2010), which has been sitting alongside a recognition that past expenditure on and provision of services has been woefully insufficient (Fonagy, 2014). Being able to generate a cross-party-political consensus on the need for increased funding for young people's mental health during the 2015 general election (YoungMinds, 2015), despite campaigning within the economic paradigm of the case for 'austerity', goes some way to illustrate the magnitude of this crisis.

However, this appreciation of need has also allowed for closer inspection of what is being offered and provided through current services and asking whether the present model of Child and Adolescent Mental Health Services is 'fit for purpose'. The previous Minister for Health and Social Care, Norman Lamb, talked about the need for a total overhaul of children and young people's mental health services, highlighting the sense of chaos and 'dysfunction' that can exist in commissioning these services. Many of the services provided are felt to be 'working in the dark ages', while others are simply unable to cope with and address demand (Press Association, 2014).

For many of the years I have been involved in Child and Adolescent Mental Health Services there have been two key issues that have repeatedly been raised regarding the provision of services for young people. Firstly, the often-heard comment about how young people 'fail to engage' with services and subsequently are discharged. Services often think about what the barriers to accessing care may be for young people – barriers such as mental health stigma – and yet seldom does one hear a more self-reflective question – such as, 'what are we actually asking these children, young people and their families to engage with?' Mental health stigma is an important and significant barrier to enabling families to access support and services, and campaigns such as Time to Change[1] have been invaluable in creating opportunities for these attitudes to be challenged. But services must also ensure they are offering something for these young people or their families to engage with that is sufficiently meaningful and acceptable to them so that they don't feel marginalised or even, at times, blamed.

The second issue that is often raised is the expression that some young people out there are too 'hard to reach'. While many may find it hard to engage with services, this is seldom because they are 'hard to reach'. We know where the young people are, but they do not feel a need for, or understand how to engage with, what is offered – especially with services offered through the statutory sector. It is clear that some of the more community-based organisations – MAC-UK,[2] with their highly innovative 'street therapy' approach – are able to work with some (although not all) of these young people, and lessons need to be learnt about practice and approach to ensure need can be addressed.

It is therefore with recognition of this wider context – a context that is as much political and economic as it is social and psychological – that, through this chapter, I shall seek to offer a perspective of practice that I believe needs to be more embedded within the community when seeking to address the mental health and emotional needs of children and young people. The focus will be on those who struggle to access what is currently on offer, outlining interventions and approaches hoping to overcome these barriers. It has been this search for such interventions that has driven my own journey as a young people's psychiatrist embedded within an outreach team. Outreach work has allowed me the space (geographically and mentally) to test out and develop ideas and ways of working – exploring what is or might be possible. But it has also reinforced my belief that most child and adolescent mental health services could be offering a practice that is much more about 'reaching out' – reaching out and being more embedded within the community.

Community, what community?

But what do I mean by practice in the community – as community has so many different meanings to different people? I am suggesting this is more than just practice that occurs outside the walls of the CAMHS clinic. It is therefore not about offering more counsellors in schools, or moving CAMHS clinicians into GP surgeries – although these initiatives have a clear impact and are not to be discouraged. Rather I am thinking about community in a much more fluid perspective – being aware that people migrate between different communities on a day-by-day, hour-by-hour basis.

With the expansion of social media and online resources, communities can also fluctuate from the global to the local at the press of a button. But communities are most importantly about where people feel they belong. Within services we often remain fixed on an idea of community being about our schools or GP surgeries, about the policeman on the beat or about dropping in to the local children's centre. But for many, and especially for those within more socio-economically deprived parts of the country, the idea of a community can be more immediate – it is focused on life on an estate, or in the stairwell, or playing basketball in the cage. The work of Lisa McKenzie (McKenzie 2015) describing life on the St Ann's estate in Nottingham highlights this understanding about community, and about where and how people feel they belong. But it also reminds us of how far services need to go if they are to be accessible to a community. There is often a suspicion, which can have some justification, of statutory services within some communities, and these suspicions need to be thought about and addressed if we are to find ways of engaging young people and families. Reaching out into communities is therefore not only about moving out of the clinic but it is also about really understanding the communities we are seeking to work within and alongside.

Unaddressed need: Exploring the inequalities, locating the barriers

With three children in every classroom (of 30) in the country having an identifiable and diagnosable mental health need (Green et al., 2004), there is clearly a huge amount of unmet, unaddressed and undetected need within all communities (Haringey Council 2014). Even if this need were to be realised and identified, services would simply be unable to cope. But even when need is noticed, there are often profound inequalities amongst those who are able to access support, which clearly needs to be considered when looking to re-configure and re-design services.

Look at the figures of males and females engaging with specific services within a community. It is readily established that more boys have mental health problems between the ages of 11 and 15 years than girls, 13% compared to 10% (Hagell et al., 2013), and yet when looking at the percentages of young people who access specific services, these figures are seldom replicated. Many young people's mental health teams will be working with up to 80% of their caseload being female. This gender imbalance is reinforced even further when one sees that these figures are reversed for young people engaged with the local youth offending services. If we are to honestly address the needs of the community, then we need to understand why it is that females are more likely to access mental health services, while males are more likely to go down the youth justice pathway.

This is not to say that all offending behaviour is about unaddressed mental health need, but when one looks at the findings from papers such as 'Nobody Made the Connection' by the Children's Commissioner (Hughes et al., 2012), one clearly sees the impact of failing to identify and address need – and, in particular, neurodevelopmental need – at an early stage. This paper highlights the far higher incidence of neurodevelopmental conditions (such as ADHD, autistic spectrum disorders or speech and language difficulties) amongst those young people who end up in young offender institutions compared to the general population. Amongst the general population, autistic spectrum difficulties are thought to present between 0.6–1.2%, but in the population of youth offender institutions the rate is estimated at 15% – a huge disparity, clearly demonstrating the need for earlier identification and intervention for these young people and their families, and also for registering the impact that this early identification might have on the wider community.

Likewise, the paper 'Talking Taboos' (YoungMinds 2012) spelt out how young people, parents and professionals feel about the issue of self-harm and how best to support young people presenting with this sign of distress. Findings showed that *only 1 in 10 young people would feel comfortable about seeking advice from a teacher, parent or GP*, and this finding was further compounded by the admission that *1 in 3 parents would not seek professional help if their child was self-harming... as many felt it reflected failure parenting or an inability to provide support at home.*

Both these papers clearly show the need to provide more appropriate, meaningful and accessible support for children, young people and their parents – while ensuring support is provided early enough to have a positive impact (Department of Health 2015).

Stepping out: Developing the right tools

My own journey in exploring and developing a community-based approach to practice was perhaps most assisted by the Targeted Mental Health in Schools project (TaMHS) (Public Health England 2012). Up until the launch of this initiative by the Department for Children, Schools and Families, my practice had developed entirely within an outreach team. Young people and families might be seen at schools, at home or other community settings, but this was often driven by needing to ensure engagement and minimising risk in cases where there was considerable concern. Previous articles (Barnes, 2012 and Barnes, 2015) have talked about how an outreach approach allows the clinician the space work alongside a young person and provides the opportunity to 'bear witness' to the experiences of these families, challenging the belief that therapy is the preserve of the clinic as working with a young person or their family over the kitchen table can be just as effective, if not more so, in building a therapeutic alliance.

But TaMHS provided both the funding and the scope for testing out ideas and initiatives with and alongside schools that has informed the development of further community interventions. But it was also the experience of working with young people for 15 years within the voluntary youth sector movement[3] that gave me the confidence and belief that things could be done differently.

For too long I had been involved in clinic-based practice where I had seen young people and their families being referred to CAMHS where they (either the young person and/or parents) felt that they were being blamed, and possibly punished, for their behaviour. Through involvement in voluntary youth sector work, it was possible to witness the impact of positive activities – from regular group nights to residentials – on young people. These opportunities create safe spaces for young people to grow and develop.

Hence, TaMHS offered the opportunity to apply this learning and experience into a community-based approach for young people's mental health services. TaMHS facilitated this stepping out of the clinic and reaching out into the community – regardless of severity of need.

Scaffolded practice

As this approach within the community was not focused on the more established outreach model of practice, it required a marked shift in perspective and approach. As noted before, the outreach approach within CAMHS is often very directed by assessment and diagnosis, with outreach interventions then being more focused on containment and crisis management. What TaMHS facilitated was an approach more reflective of community psychological interventions and therefore needed the appropriate tools and framework.

An opportunity to work and train in Cognitive Analytic Therapy (CAT)[4] provided some of the psychological tools needed to ensure that the support offered through this 'reaching out' was sufficiently scaffolded to feel safe and robust. I should stress I am not suggesting that CAT is the only therapeutic training that could offer a containing framework for understanding and working within the community. But the appeal of CAT is its collaborative approach to engagement and its integrative theory which allows for a more relational approach to mental health (Potter 2015). Many young people and parents find a CAT-based approach helpful, feeling they are working alongside the clinician, not relying entirely on 'talking' but also being able to access diagrams, draw maps or write letters as ways of gaining insight into their difficulties. It is also an approach that is easily adapted to the setting – from mapping on the streets (Potter, 2010) to therapeutic self-harm assessments (Ougrin, 2010). At the same time, the CAT model has an evolving evidence base in working with young people with significant mental health needs within the community as highlighted by interventions such as the *Helping Young People Early* (HYPE) model developed by Orygen Youth Health in Melbourne (Chanen et al., 2013).

But it is also some of the theoretical underpinnings of CAT – and in particular the work of Vygotsky that felt most helpful when exploring this community-based practice – building on Vygotsky's concept of the zone of proximal development (ZPD), and the educational construct of scaffolded learning (Illeris, 2009). The ZPD can be defined as *'the gap between what a child is able to do alone and what he/she could learn to do with the provision of appropriate help from a more competent other, be they parent, teacher or peer'* (Ryle et al., 2002). But, fundamentally I see working in the ZPD being about working where the young person *is at*, rather than where others would like them to *be at.*

Building on working in the ZPD, and ensuring practice was sufficiently supported and scaffolded, facilitated a move away from the clinic: a reaching out and enabling practice within the community.

Stepping out: Applying theory into practice

Armed with a theoretical framework to underpin community practice, it has been possible to develop a number of projects and initiatives that have enabled this reaching out from clinic-based practice. When thinking about working with young people, and wanting to be working where they 'are at', then, for some, this is football! But building on this rather well-established observation, in combination with the necessary psychological tools, it was possible to develop a therapeutically informed programme, *A Game of 2 Halves* (www. rcpsych.ac.uk 2014), based on the dialogue and involvement that can be accessed through football.

Evolving into a 12-week programme for young people at risk of exclusion from school, this group initiative supported students to develop emotional literacy skills, promoted self-regulation and mentalisation and built their resilience. But, most importantly, it was all delivered through a dialogue and engagement with football.

In reality, the programme has little to do with football – rather it is about allowing football to be the tool and vehicle for engagement. This type of programme could just have easily been about dance or drama or cooking. The model can also be easily adapted and has been transferred to other settings, such as pupil referral units, youth offending services or working on estates. There are programmes up and down the country that offer similar interventions in many different settings.[5] What matters is creating a setting that will appeal, that will allow young people to feel safe and to connect, hence facilitating engagement. The right tools for engagement are essential to engage the right groups, but there needs to be a clear framework and thinking surrounding the intervention that allows for genuine opportunities for change. This is not simply about letting a group of young people go off and play football, but it is about using football to provide the space for relationships to develop and for trust to be established, which eventually allows the space for change.

Similar thinking is required when young people struggle to engage with what is offered. *K.Dot* was a film made by a group of students following the death of their friend outside a chicken shop at the end of the school day. These friends found themselves confronting loss and trauma when they should have been able to focus on their studies. Not surprisingly the whole school was devastated, and support was offered from within the school as well as from agencies outside – with the shock and distress impacting far across the community. But it was as school life started to get back on track, as most of the students felt able to start moving forwards, without feeling they were letting down their friend or colleague, that the impact on this closer group of friends started to emerge.

These friends gradually became more and more disengaged from school, from their families and perhaps even from 'life' as they struggled to make sense of losing their friend. Services – from CAMHS to social care, from educational psychology to youth offending services – all sought to offer support to these young people and their families, but little was taken up. Whatever was on offer just didn't appear to resonate with this group.

The group were eventually invited to produce a film as a tribute to their friend – and hence the creation of the film *K.Dot* (Baker 2012). Shown on a snowy January evening to a packed school auditorium, friends and family saw a group of young people talk on screen through the stages of their grief and loss as they came to terms with the passing of their friend. The making of a film, along with mentoring support and supervision for the delivery team, allowed this group the chance to reflect and the space to process what had occurred to their friend. It also gave them the time to think about what had been going on for themselves since and it proved a turning point for most as they found ways to reconnect with their education and learning.

But having appreciated the wider impact of this trauma on the whole school community, alongside the reception of the *K.Dot* film, then the opportunity to explore ways of working through a whole-school approach, looking to address need across the wider school community, seemed the obvious next step, and allowed for the evolution of Time 2 Talk.

Time 2 Talk[6] is an award-winning project that aimed to raise awareness and understanding about mental and emotional well-being amongst the whole school community – students, staff and parents. But it also looked to challenge the stigma regarding self-harm, mental health and emotional distress and bring about lasting systemic change in approach and process for addressing the mental health needs within the school. It allowed a journey to evolve through narratives and drama, through filmmaking and lesson planning, through peer mentoring and staff training, so that eventually the whole school community had had the opportunity to be involved. This project offered both a preventative and early-help approach, and sits alongside other whole-school approaches that seek to build resilience within the whole school community (Hart et al., 2007). But it is also building upon a growing evidence base for the effectiveness and importance of wider school-based approaches – approaches that are now being shown to have an impact on high-risk mental-health need such as suicidal ideation (Wassermann et al., 2015).

Towards a relational approach to mental health

Although the projects outlined offer differing perspectives and ways of approaching need within the community/ies, there is one common thread that holds them all together. For it is the quality of the 'helping relationship' – either between peer mentor and student, between student and teacher, between mentor and group, between football coach and team, or between parent and child – that, in the end, determines the effectiveness of such support.

We know that services are currently unable to address the total level of need, and this is likely to remain the case for some time, and therefore we need to find alternative means of support – either in school, online or in estates. We need to enable young people to support each other, to empower parents to feel able to support each other to help manage their child's upset and distress and to provide teachers with the understanding and tools to offer enough to students to help build resilience. But this is not about displacing responsibility from services. Rather it should be seen as acknowledging that communities perhaps have felt undermined in recent years with clinical experts being consulted – perhaps at the price of dismissing expertise and experience that already exists within the community.

Peer mentoring offers a potential solution to addressing some of this increased need. Structured mentoring programmes that focus on positive youth development models seem to promote increased levels of emotional resilience in both the mentor and mentee (Dubois et al., 2002), resulting in positive impacts on health, educational attendance and attainment as well as offending behaviours. But these models need to focus on the development of the interpersonal relationship as well as thinking about the socio-emotional development and cognitive development to be effective. Recent collaborative ventures such as the More than Mentors (Brown 2015) programme in the London Borough of Newham have sought to explore some of the evidence for this type of intervention as they are often a better starting place for some, and certainly more accessible than being referred to a clinic.

The model of mentoring/peer mentoring has previously been strongly associated with education, and offered primarily to improve attendance and attainment. But there is an emerging appreciation (Department for Education 2015) that this approach – of peer-to-peer support – is enabling and empowering for all, including peer-support parenting programmes, which show strong evidence of impact.[7]

For if we are to provide opportunities for young people to change, or even space for mutual support, then we need to ensure there is a capacity to build and develop trust. Interventions that seek to build epistemic trust[8] such as the Adolescent Mentalisation-Based Integrative Treatment (AMBIT),[9] provide a genuine way of connecting with young people with significant attachment difficulties. Even more refreshingly, this approach doesn't rely on a single speciality holding an exclusive understanding of the young person's emotional distress, but allows a more holistic perspective of the young person to be considered – allowing thinking together to be fostered across teams, networks and services, which also generates an awareness of the benefits of integration. The community-based approaches developed by the integrate model[10] highlight the opportunity for building sustainable relationships with mentors or key-workers that can be supported and sustained by professionals in the 'team around the keyworker' – providing services with the opportunity to work collaboratively, efficiently and effectively rather than in isolation (Gilburt et al., 2014).

But if we can start to create the space for young people to support each other, then we have an opportunity to move away from the stance of failing to address the needs of those who 'do not engage' with services, or ignore those who are felt to be 'hard to reach'. Those who have previously been unable to access support in clinic-based services can access support – but this support needs to be offered where they 'are at', both developmentally and with regard to locality.

Reaching out and embedding practice in the community: Less about choice and more about necessity

If we seriously want to address the growing mental health needs of young people then we really need to consider what we are providing to address this need, as well as consider how we might prevent the need arising in the first place. What I have discussed in this chapter offers nothing new – it is simply a request that we broaden our gaze – moving away from what is on offer in the clinic and thinking more about where young people 'are at' within their communities.

Fundamentally I feel we need to remind ourselves what it is we are seeking to provide. We want to offer opportunities for change for some young people and their families – while at the same time we want to offer guidance and support to help communities support each other to manage distress and difficulties at an earlier stage. However, to achieve this we need to hand over some of the 'intellectual authority' that can be assumed within clinical/specialised services. After all, there are many more experts by experience within the community than there are CAMHS clinicians.

We all want our young people to grow up healthy and resilient – to cope with some of the difficulties that life will throw at them, but also knowing when to reach out and ask for help. Young people need to be able to trust those around them and can only do this through experiencing positive relationships. We therefore need a perspective of mental health that is positive and seen as everyone's business rather than just the remit of the specialist in the CAMHS clinic. But this is why practice has to move out of the clinic. Remaining solely in the clinic is about maintaining distance and reinforcing barriers. But armed with an understanding of a relational approach to mental health and equipped with tools that allow us all to work where young people 'are at' – we have a far better chance of addressing the 'national crisis' that is young people's mental health. Reaching out and embedding practice in the community is less of a choice and more of a necessity.

Notes

[1] Time to Change. Further information available at www.time-to-change.org.uk/

[2] Music and Change (MAC-UK). Further information available at www.mac-uk.org/

[3] Voluntary Youth Sector work through groups such as the International Falcon Movement. Further information available at www.ifm-sei.org/ and Woodcraft Folk – further information available at woodcraft.org.uk

[4] Cognitive Analytic Therapy (CAT). Further information available at www.acat.me.uk/page/home

[5] Such as Football beyond Borders. Further information available at www.footballbeyondborders.org/

[6] Time 2 Talk, winner of the HSJ Awards 2015: Innovation in mental health, 18th November 2015. Available at www.hsj.co.uk/more/awards/hsj-awards/hsj-awards-2015-innovation-in-mental-health/7000296.fullarticle

[7] EPEC – Empowering parents, empowering communities. More information available at www.cpcs.org.uk/index.php?page=empowering-parents-empowering-communities

[8] Epistemic Trust – definition available at ambit-content.tiddlyspace.com/ Epistemic%20Trust

[9] Adolescent Mentalisation Based Integrative Treatment (AMBIT). More information available at http://ambit.tiddlyspace.com/

[10] The Integrate Model. More information available at www.mac-uk.org/ integrate/the-integrate-model/

References

Baker, H. (2012). Friends of murdered Tottenham teenager Kasey Gordon get lottery grant for knife crime film project. 12th May 2012, *Haringey Independent* (Online). Available at www.haringeyindependent.co.uk/ news/9701368.Friends_of_murdered_teenager_Kasey_Gordon_get_ lottery_grant_for_knife_crime_film/ (Accessed 2nd October 2015).

Barnes, N. (2012). Context 120. Outreach – Reaching out in different contexts, April 2012.

Barnes, N. (2015). Reformulation, Issue 45. Winter, 2015. Reaching Out – A Journey Within and Alongside CAT.

Brown, J. (2015). Peer Mentoring Plan Set to Boost Mental Health in Schools. Children and Young People Now, 10-23 November 2015. Further information about More than Mentors. Available at www. uclpartners.com/news/pilot-project-awarded-newham/, (Accessed 4 September 2015).

Chanen, A. and McCutcheon, L. (2013). Prevention and early intervention for borderline personality disorder: current status and recent evidence. *British Journal of Psychiatry*, 202 s24–s29.

Collishaw, S., Maughan, B., Natarajan, L. and Pickles, A. (2010). Trends in adolescent emotional problems in England: A comparison of two national cohorts twenty years apart. *Journal of Child Psychology and Psychiatry*, 51, 8, 885–894. Also quoted in Nuffield Foundation (2013), Changing Adolescence Programme briefing paper. Social trends and mental health: introducing the main findings.

Cooper, C. (2014). Exclusive: Children's mental healthcare in crisis, Care Minister Norman Lamb admits. *The Independent* (Online) 20th August. Available at www.independent.co.uk/life-style/health-and-families/ health-news/exclusive-childrens-mental-healthcare-in-crisis-care-minister- norman-lamb-admits-9679098.html (Accessed 4th October 2015).

Department for Education (2015). Minister for Childcare and Education, Sam Gyimah (MP) outlines existing and planned work on mental health in schools. First presented on 3rd December 2015. Available at www.gov.uk/government/speeches/

children-and-young-peoples-mental-health-in-schools?utm_
source=twitterfeed&utm_medium=twitter

Department of Health (2015). Future in mind – Promoting, protecting
and improving our children and young people's mental health and
wellbeing (Online). The Children and Young People's Mental Health
and Wellbeing Taskforce. Available at www.gov.uk/government/uploads/
system/uploads/attachment_data/file/414024/Childrens_Mental_Health.
pdf (Accessed 2nd October 2015).

DuBois, D.L., Holloway, B.E., Valentine, J.C. and Cooper, H. (2002).
Effectiveness of mentoring programs for youth: a meta-analytic review. *Am
J Community Psychol*, 30(2):157–97.

Fonagy, P, (2014). Children and Young People's Improved Access to
Psychological Therapies Newsletter (Online). April. Available at www.
cypiapt.org/site-files/Newsletter%20April%202014%20Final.pdf
(Accessed 2nd October 2015).

Gilburt, H., Edwards, N. and Murray, R. (2014). Transforming mental
health – A plan of action for London, 25 September 2014. The Kings
Fund. Available at www.kingsfund.org.uk/publications/transforming-
mental-health (Accessed 2nd October 2015).

Green, H., McGinnity, A., Meltzer, H. et al. (2004). Mental health of
children and young people in Great Britain 2004, Summary report.
Published 31st August 2005. National Statistics (online). Available at
www.hscic.gov.uk/pubs/mentalhealth04 (Accessed 2nd October 2015).

Hagell, A., Coleman, J. and Brooks, F. (2013). Key data on Adolescence.
London, Association for Young People's health. Available at www.ayph.
org.uk/publications/457_AYPH_KeyData2013_WebVersion.pdf, (Accessed
26th July 2015).

Haringey Council (2014). Annual Public Health Report, How good are
we feeling? Wellbeing and poor mental health (Online). Available at
www.haringey.gov.uk/sites/haringeygovuk/files/how_good_are_we_
feeling_2014-2.pdf. (Accessed 2nd October 2015).

Hart, A. and Blincow, D. (2007). Available at www.boingboing.org.uk/
index.php/resilience-in-practice/what-is-resilient-therapy (Accessed 2nd
October 2015).

Hughes, N., Williams, H., Chitsabesan, P., Davies, R. and Mounce, L. (2012).
Nobody made a connection: The prevalence of neurodisability in young
people who offend, October, Children's Commissioner. Table 1{{{citation
type=tb idref=tb1 }}}. The prevalence of neurodevelopmental disorders,
page 23. Available at www.childrenscommissioner.gov.uk/sites/default/
files/publications/Nobody%20made%20the%20connection.pdf
(Accessed 2nd October 2015).

Illeris, K. (ed.) (2009). *Contemporary Theories of Learning: Learning Theorists ...
In Their Own Words, Routledge*. Abingdon, Oxon.

Mckenzie, L. (2015). *Estates, Class and Culture in Austerity Britain Policy*, Press University of Bristol.

Press Association (2014) Child mental health services 'stuck in the dark ages', says Norman Lamb. *The Guardian* (online). Available at www.theguardian.com/society/2014/aug/20/child-mental-health-dark-ages-norman-lamb. (Accessed 2nd October 2015).

Ougrin, D., Zundel, T. and Ng, A. (2010). *Self-Harm Assessment in Young People – A Therapeutic Assessment Manual*. Hodder Arnold, London.

Potter, S. (2010). Words with Arrows – The Benefits of Mapping Whilst Talking. *Reformulation*, Summer, pp. 37–45.

Potter, S. (2015). What do we mean by Relational Mental Health? International Cognitive Analytic Therapy Association (online) Available at http://internationalcat.org/relational-mental-health-the-cognitive-analytic-contribution/ (Accessed 2nd October 2015).

Public Health England, National Child and Maternal Health Intelligence Network (2012). Targeting Mental Health in Schools final evaluation (2008–2011) (online) Available at www.chimat.org.uk/camhs/tamhs/eval (Accessed 2nd October 2015).

Royal College of Psychiatry website (2014). The 'Beautiful Game' helps support young people at risk of exclusion from school. June 2014 (online). Available at www.rcpsych.ac.uk/mediacentre/pressreleases2014/the%E2%80%98beautifulgame%E2%80%99helpssup.aspx (Accessed 2nd October 2015).

Ryle, A. and Kerr, I. (2002). *Introducing Cognitive Analytic Therapy: Principles and Practice*. Wiley. p41. Hoboken, New Jersey USA.

Wassermann, D. et al. (2015). School-based suicide prevention programmes: the SEYLE cluster-randomised, controlled. Lancet - Volume 385, No. 9977, p1536–1544, 18 April 2015. Available at www.thelancet.com/journals/lancet/article/PIIS0140-6736(14)61213-7/fulltext (Accessed 2nd October 2015).

YoungMinds (2012). Talking Taboos – Talking Self-Harm. Young Minds and Cello, 2012. Available at www.cellogroup.com/pdfs/talking_self_harm.pdf (Accessed 2nd October 2015).

YoungMinds (2015) – Available at www.youngminds.org.uk/news/blog/2730_join_our_keepyourword_campaign (Accessed 2nd October 2015).

11

'WHO CAN I TURN TO?' MAKING HEALTHCARE MORE RELATIONSHIP-CENTRED AND NOT SYSTEM-CENTRED

Sarah Campbell and Jenny Cobb

In place of a prescriptive framework, this chapter will explore and enquire with the reader what 'therapeutic' and 'relationship' means for the child, young person and frontline practitioner. Themes will be supported with illustrations drawn from research involving a service-user study (YoungMinds, 2013; Campbell, 2014) as well as appropriate practice material advocating for the young person's and practitioner's voice. The current environment within which the child and adolescent mental health service (CAMHS) sits will be introduced critically to try to better understand the strains placed on preserving the therapeutic relationship. This type of professional relationship has historically been the domain of frontline practitioners, such as mental health nurses, probation officers, specialist teachers and social workers, and has been developed and passed on generationally over the decades to offer a service to troubled children, young people and their families. Through this exploration, it is hoped that the reader will be able to recognise and define the nature of relationship-centred practice and understand the major factors involved in either sustaining or negating this essential and core professional activity for future generations of practitioners.

So far in this new millennium, there have been significant shifts in the way CAMHS have come to be thought about and how treatment, care and support is offered to infants, children and young people in England and Wales. There have been some positive contributions to shape and uphold priority, such as the policy document *Early Intervention: The Next Steps* (Allen, 2011), as growing recognition is realised in political circles that in order to promote a healthy society there have to be healthy beginnings. A context of health economics supported this realisation. However, contrary to this social development an unfortunate moment in economic history also occurred, with its impact echoing throughout all public service areas and which has been particularly apparent within mental health services. A shift of policy determined by austere fiscal planning bore witness to some clinically good intentions, similar to the content of the *Early Intervention* document (ibid), which are being let go and/or abandoned in the flood of economic panic and political manoeuvring. Other later documents such as *Future in Mind* (2015) do not extend the full potential of *Early Intervention* (ibid) but seem more derivative of 'the state we're in' with further suggestions and proposals to tackle the 'gaps in service' through better evidenced-based care. Perhaps an irony abounds here when one's colleagues have had to face a further tranche of staff cutbacks, or that training budgets have been cut by a further 25% or that the duration and diversity of some care pathways have been absolutely minimalised to manage human resource. Where do we look for the evidence base here?

We have reached a critical point where the CAMHS provision is often viewed by those wanting its service (both clinical and consultative) as inaccessible and over stretched (Coyne, 2015; Teggart and Linden, 2006). In the YoungMinds study (Campbell et al., 2013/14), many examples were given by practitioners to support the difficulty of getting adequate service provision because of the long waiting lists and how this encouraged young people to look for alternatives. Practitioners linked this directly to an increase in offending behaviour in young people.

> There is a long waiting list for CAMHS which means things like offending can get worse because no one is giving them the right attention. (Professional)

Additionally, participants in the study expressed their concern around CAMHS resourcing and the pressure on streamlining and local determining of service provision to accommodate managing CAMHS waiting lists which can carry penalties. These factors were felt to be detrimental to a comprehensive CAMH service provision.

The service seems to be increasingly dependent on diagnostic criteria as a means of justifying funding and care pathways organised to meet current policy criteria (Timimi, 2012; Rutter, 2011). This economic model of payment by results imposes a non-clinical bureaucracy that constrains rather than illuminates the real needs of service users. Elsewhere in this book, authors (Wilson, Timimi) have expressed serious concern about the convenience with which some research supports this model by contributing to an evidence base. An educated audience recognises that research can be shaped.

Has this situation alongside long waiting lists and short treatment packages contributed to a general loss of clinically credible practice? An influx of organisational changes needed to implement the austerity measures seems to have demoralised many practitioners: nobody likes to be restructured, to be asked to reapply for their job, to be told they can no longer offer the treatment, care and support for which they have spent years in training to develop appropriate skills and which makes best use of evidence-based knowledge and understanding. Although practitioners are used to adapting to 'changing' environments and understand the importance of 'fitting in', there are clinical limits to any of this, whereby the essence of the practitioner role can slip away and it simply becomes a cipher.

We only have to look towards the Francis Inquiry (2013) to see how far-reaching this system-centred practice devised from an economic business model can be destructive and damaging to the patient and to the service alike.

Additionally these alterations to service organisation and treatment provision have minimalised clinical practice opportunities where once established and robust frontline practice took place and acted as an essential training ground for our young junior practitioners. These environments were the backbone of vital training often referred to as 'learning in and from experience' (Schon, 1983; Boud, 1991). It is from such experiences as these that relationship-centred practice naturally emerges and has developed, historically sustained by robust clinical leadership and the provision of a reflective supervisory space. Higher education for professional learning is imperative and enables experienced frontline practitioners to expand their knowledge and appreciate valid research and evidence. This learning however can only make sense when the student is exposed to practice environments that are thoughtful and allow the child to be at the centre of the work.

Initially, services develop to meet a clear and identifiable need and not a budget and yet clearly professionals have to work within a viable economic context. These are often competing tensions that require practice not only to be thought about and reviewed managerially but, most importantly, clinically too.

The lived experience

It is estimated that one in five children will experience mental health difficulties within their young lives and one in ten of these children will come to the attention of a helping professional (DH, 2015).

The most comprehensive statistical survey of the prevalence of mental disorders in Great Britain found that in 2004 10% of children and young people aged between 5 and 15 had a clinically diagnosable mental disorder that is associated with 'considerable distress and substantial interference with personal functions' such as family and social relationships, their capacity to cope with day-to-day stresses and life challenges, and their learning (Green, McGinnity, Meltzer et al., 2005). Nearly one-third of children diagnosed as having emotional disorders in 2004 still had them in 2007, with family, household and social characteristics strongly linked to persistence (Parry-Langdon (ed.), 2008). Little seems to have changed.

This statistical information certainly maps out the enormity of the national problem for our policymakers to be concerned with. However, at grass roots, even if experiencing high levels of mental distress, it may take quite some time before the idea of turning to someone for help takes shape in the minds of the child or the family. But to whom do they turn and in what context?

The lived experience of children is essentially a social one and it is also within a social context that professional help is offered.

Over the past two decades, there have been numerous reports, recommendations, directives and guidance (DH, 2004a; DH, 2004b; National CAMHS Review Expert Group, 2008; DH, 2009; DH, 2012: DH, 2015) that have sought to outline, clarify, define and formally direct the frameworks for the delivery of care. These are clearly envisioned as social systems designed to improve services. Yet what is evident is that at some fundamental level within each of these frameworks there is a failure to fully address the needs of the child or young person, or realistically address the full costs of change, particularly within the social system that delivers care.

What initially starts out as a meaningful and effective (social) solution to providing a rational, qualitative and quantifiable service of care may quickly become a problem in practice (Barker 2009).

What is the missing element within these frameworks? Listening to what children and young people and their families say, it is the vital recognition of the profound and compounding complexities of the lived realities of their lives – and with a developmental trajectory that will last well until the child's or young person's mid-twenties: what really may be required in terms of the help provided?

Through the YoungMinds study (Campbell et al., 2014), young people and practitioners spoke about their referrals to CAMHS frequently not meeting rigid criteria and high thresholds and if they were, the referral pathway was often blocked. If they received a referral and saw a professional, the most common experience young people had of mental health services related to the prescribing and taking of medication. While for some young people the medication helped, for others the consequences of the side effects were far reaching.

> *The medication they put me on, it was making me that drained and I was dribbling all the time, I couldn't even care for my son. That's why I had to send my son to his dad's … its affected my life even more losing him, really. (YP8)*

Some young people interviewed showed an awareness of debates about the appropriateness of prescribing medication to younger people. One had wanted medication but was denied it. Two others felt that their medication needed a review, but found it difficult to get one.

> *I'm trying to say, look, my medication needs to be looked at all the time, you can't just give it me and then leave me for two years. It needs to be moderated, we need to look at it, make sure that it's still working. Because this was the problem that I had with the medication before, which is why I stopped taking it, because it wasn't working … (YP2)*

It is these very complexities that thoroughly test professional abilities, service resources and provisions as well as accurately identifying future needs. The two social systems (that of the family and that of the service provider) can be antithetical and this has consequences. The patients' voice, captured through service user research, has conveyed these messages within several reports (Coyne, 2015; Hovish, 2012; Worrall-Davies, 2008; Teggart and Linden, 2006) yet the directions pursued by policy frameworks demonstrate that there are real difficulties in translating this into service provision.

Arising from the Francis Inquiry (ibid) the drive to make care provision more human-centred places a focus on social systems to put people and the personal at the heart of care delivery. It challenges professionals to deliver care in a human-centred way that truly promotes and fosters relationships.

But for the child and family, it is this capacity to relate and their experience of relationships that can become so adversely affected at times of emotional disturbances (whatever its root) and it is therefore a real, legitimate need of the child, or his/her family, to be able to turn to professionals who *can* relate and sustain relationships effectively. The following excerpt (YoungMinds, 2013) reveals how discontinuity and disrupted relationships with staff made the building of helpful therapeutic relationships difficult.

> *My problem is opening up to people I don't know. I like to work with the same person all the time because once I've met that person, you know me, I know you, there's no need for 23 introductions and then each time I work with them I get to know them a bit better, so by the end we've got a good rapport. But I don't want to have to keep being thrown to and from this person, that person. (YP2)*

A major emphasis within the data was the lack of staff continuity. YP1, for example, reported having had six different professionals in three months.

With this in mind, it would seem essential that professional practice has at its very core a service delivery model that fully facilitates this: a relationship-centred model of intervention and care. This message was clearly outlined in the Munro Review (2011) proposals for reform, which, taken together, are intended to create conditions that enable professionals, social workers in particular, to make the best judgments about the help to give children, young people and families. The review suggests moving from a system that has become over-bureaucratised and focused on compliance to one that values and develops professional expertise and is focused on the safety and welfare of children and young people.

To hear another voice from a young person who started to offend after the death of his father and whose participation in the study really identifies that when professionals (in this case, school staff) do not listen, the results can be so damaging.

> *They never sat down and said to me, what is the problem? They never took up the issue of my dad dying and of giving me that sympathy, or not even just the sympathy, they never gave me the time to even grieve. They just wanted me to do exams and exams, exams and they never took it into consideration that I was grieving for my father. (YP12)*

Children and young people face a highly complex, social world, one constantly changing and in a state of flux: one that offers unparalleled opportunities as well as threats. A world wherein relating and relationships can be everyday and at times, painfully all too real, or indeed be virtual and anonymous. Professionals too are working in similarly highly complex service delivery systems and one of the repeated recommendations to emerge from findings is the need for professionals to think about their work within a reflective supervisory space.

Clinical supervision within the helping professions particularly within mental health and social care has been seen over several decades as essential in supporting professional development and learning (Fowler, 1996; Cutcliffe, Butterworth and Proctor, 2001; Brunero and Stein-Parbury, 2007).

Scott Brunero and Jane Stein-Parbury describe the activity within nursing:

> The primary cognitive process of clinical supervision is reflection, that is, thinking back on clinical experiences in order to recount them and deepen understanding ... Reflection is particularly relevant to professional growth in a practice-based discipline such as nursing. That is, nursing knowledge is embedded in experience, and learning through experience is essential to the practice of professional nursing. (Brunero and Stein-Parbury, 2007 p87)

However, despite the findings and recommendations of the Francis Report and Munro Review it appears less acknowledged by frontline services that clinical supervision is a vital part of patient/service-user care. In times when services are being asked to creatively look at treatment and care models that reduce resources, it is perhaps even more imperative to appreciate the impact and function of appropriate clinical supervision in the treatment, care and support of troubled children, young people and families.

Interestingly, research conducted by Bradshaw, Butterworth and Mairs (2007) within in-patient adult mental health services assessed whether clinical supervision provided by workplace-based supervisors can enhance outcomes for mental health nurses and the service users with whom they work. This study found that service users seen by the nurses in the experimental group showed significantly greater reductions in positive psychotic symptoms and total symptoms compared with those seen by nurses in the control group. It is disappointing and curious that in an era where practice-based research supports the evidence base used to dictate policy and procedure there is a noticeable dearth of similar studies representing all clinical areas.

Minds at work: Thinking about relationships

Ongoing supervised practice is a touchstone of the professional relationship, and yet we know that in reality supervision of practise fails to be implemented or sustained across much of service provision (White and Winstanley, 2012; Bradshaw and Butterworth, 2007; Cutcliffe, Butterworth and Proctor, 2001). Managerial and/or professional supervision is more widely implemented than is supervision of actual practice.

While CAMH services have been more likely to provide professionals with the space for clinical supervision and training, other sectors, such as education services (which now have a major remit in monitoring child mental health) have little or no tradition. But even in CAMH services, recent changes suggest, here too provision can be patchy and inconsistent (DH 2013). This is also reflected in supporting practitioners gaining higher education which offers a vital space to critique the evidence and develop professionally.

One clear way a service provider has of maintaining a relationship-centred approach is to never knowingly underestimate the complexity of the child and family's life, nor the complexities of its own service provision and the impact one has on the other. A space to think is required at all levels within an organisation not just by those directly engaged with the child or family.

When thinking about these complexities, Figure 11.1 schematically draws the child at the centre of its own life, shaping and being shaped by his/her own internal and external worlds and this presents real challenges to the professional: to know and to understand what may be going on for that child.

Whatever areas of a child's life the professional focuses upon, there will always be unknown factors present – aspects not readily accessible or available to know. Even when significant information may be known about a child or family, as many professionals are aware, it is still very helpful to find a way of maintaining a stance of 'open enquiry' that is a curiosity and a willingness to learn more. This can be a difficult position for a professional to both hold and maintain given the demands for expert assessment, diagnosis, intervention and the requirement of contracts as well as the need to meet specific targets. As Eileen Munro (2008) states, the single most

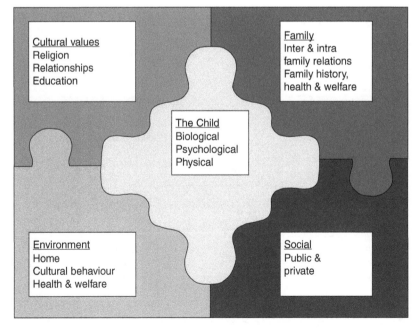

Figure 11.1

important factor in minimising errors is to be able to think, reflect and admit that you may be wrong.

The professional is also required to hold in mind his/her own social system (Figure 11.2). While using available theories and developmental models of mind as well as researched best practices and outcomes in an up-to-date way, the professional holds onto her/his understanding of the service and wider professional social systems in which (s)he practises. It is imperative that given this complexity, a safe space called supervision is made available to distil this and to discuss and think about their experiences with a child and family.

This stance is endorsed, perhaps only too painfully, by the NSPCC's Case Reviews (NSPCC, 2013, 2014, 2015). These reviews highlight the degree to which professionals are working both in and across highly complex social systems, including the child's own, and in its overview of recommendations arising from its case reviews, the NSPCC concurs that supervision is an essential cornerstone of practice and that it should assist practitioners with the discipline of reflective thinking (NSPCC, 2014, 2015).

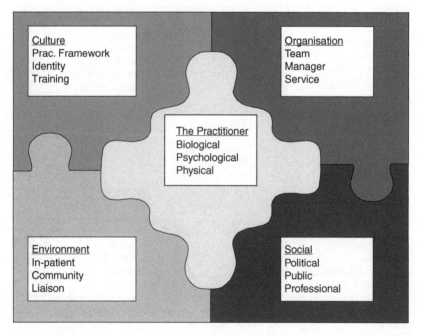

Figure 11.2

A simple example, drawn from an acute environment indicates the question of need.

A young female mental health nurse has her ankle and shin stroked by a male young person on the unit. The nurse giggles and moves away to a different part of the unit. She manages the situation by avoiding this patient in the subsequent week.

The questions this scenario raises are many: Why did the nurse giggle? Why did the nurse use avoidance as a strategy? How does this represent a therapeutic relationship? What was the young person communicating through his action? It is through a carefully facilitated supervisory discussion that a deeper understanding for the nurse can be explored and realised: a real 'learning from experience' can occur. This new depth of understanding and thinking empowers her to take up a different stronger more confident position with this young person without having to fall back on avoidance strategies. This may offer the young person a therapeutic opportunity through a relationship-centred practice approach and a knowledge somewhere that there is a team holding him in mind and responding to his need for treatment in a thoughtful way. We can see from this simple example that the impact the work has on the practitioner cannot be underestimated and requires time for consideration. This can only be achieved through strong leadership and skilful supervision, without which the opportunity to work therapeutically as a practitioner is compromised and the system of care moves into an area of knee-jerk reactions that diminishes therapeutic relationships encouraging poor decision making through a weakened professional stance.

Working in a relationship-centred way with a child or family is not easy. The child may be deeply troubled and the whole family highly disturbed by its experiences. The work is challenging, painful, anxiety-provoking and often the greatest fear is of becoming overwhelmed by it all. Without the containment provided by supervision and training, the professional may be subtly pushed or pulled away from maintaining a therapeutic position.

The space provided by supervision can also promote thinking about the myriad of social systems operating at any given time in the child's life as well as the professional's. For some children their experiences of hurt, loss, uncertainty, disadvantage and deprivation are repeated yet again within the service of care they receive (Read et al., 1996; Schmidt Neven, 2010).

For example, when leaving the care system, young people report that they can encounter a significant recapitulation of much earlier adverse experiences, and feel unprepared, uncertain and unsupported (Green, 2005; DH, 2013). Or children may feel an abandonment when services discharge them precipitously because the child's family does not, or cannot engage, or when a service is unable to grasp the true seriousness or precariousness of the child's circumstances.

In the YoungMinds Report (Campbell et al., 2013/14), professionals expressed concern that the legal status of 'intentionally homeless' reduces options and precipitates further offending behaviour, criminalising young people. These young people often come from high-risk and abusive backgrounds, which are traumatic and precipitated them being 'in need' and 'in care'.

> And a lot of the behaviours, particularly around offending, also around things like becoming 'intentionally homeless' through housing law, start closing doors for your future at that age. And for people, for example, leaving care, fine, I'm homeless on my 18th birthday, that's good, isn't it, because I've blown, got an arson offence, ... and I've been kicked out of three hostels, therefore I'm intentionally homeless. May as well say, 'OK, youth offending institute's over there, your honour, just walk to the gate and admit yourself', because unfortunately that's where a lot of them (care leavers) are going. (Professional)

While practise supervision and professional education can and will help the professional address these kinds of experiences with colleagues and with children and families, the Francis Report (2013) is taking a wider 'whole-systems' approach in its recommendation that organisations providing care should '...create and maintain the right culture to deliver high-quality care that is responsive to patients' needs and preferences'.

The delivery of the level and complexity of services that children and their families require in the 21st century – within a culture that remains steadfastly human-centred in how it operates – remains an ongoing challenge.

The challenge lies in addressing the costs that such a cultural change requires. These costs are as multifaceted as they are considerable. So while the hope is for a positive cultural change, wherein the space for thinking is provided through readily available and accessible supervision of practise and higher education, it is set against this other backdrop – that of the current trajectory of the NHS. This vital social system, that at its very core holds the most dependent and vulnerable of all in our society, also needs help.

As highlighted in its publication *Closing the Gap: Better Value Health Care for Patients* (Monitor 2012) it will require everyone's effort to ensure that the NHS can deliver what it needs to deliver deep into the 21st century and beyond

This notion of relationship goes far beyond that articulated in the Francis Report (2013) or suggested within the Future in Mind report (2015) and sets us all an even greater test in ensuring that when a child or young person experiencing mental distress asks 'who can I turn to?' there is an ongoing responsive and effective reply.

References

Appleby, J. Galea, A. and Murray, R. (2014). *The NHS Productivity Challenge: Experience from the Front Line.* London: The King's Fund.

Bone, C. (2015). '"They're not witches. ..." Young children and their parents' perceptions and experiences of Child and Adolescent Mental Health Services'. *Child care, health and development (0305–1862),* 41 (3), p. 450.

Boud, D.J. and Walker, D. (1991). *Experience and Learning: Reflection at Work.* Victoria: Deakon University.

Boud, D., Cressey, P. and Docherty, P. (eds) (2006). *Productive Reflection at Work: Learning for Changing Organisations.* London: Routledge.

Bradshaw, T., Butterworth, A. and Mairs, H. (2007). Does structured clinical supervision during psychosocial intervention education enhance outcome for mental health nurses and the service users they work with? *Journal of Psychiatric and Mental Health Nursing* 14 (1), 4–12.

Brunero, S. and Stein-Parbury, J. (2008). The effectiveness of clinical supervision in nursing: An evidenced based literature review. *Australian Journal of Advanced Nursing.* 25 (3), 86–94.

Campbell, S. Simpson, A. and Abbot, S. (2014). 'Young offenders with mental health problems in transition'. *The Journal of Mental Health Training, Education, and Practice (1755-6228),* 9 (4), 232.

Coyne, I., McNamara, N., Healy, M., Gower, C., Sarkar, M. and McNicholas, F. (2015). Adolescents' and parents' views of Child and Adolescent Mental Health Services (CAMHS) in Ireland. *Journal of Psychiatric and Mental Health Nursing,* 22, 561–569. doi: 10.1111/jpm.12215

Cutcliffe, John R., Butterworth, T. and Proctor, B (2001) *Fundamental Themes in Clinical Supervision.* London: Routledge.

Department of Health (1990a). *Caring for People. The Care Programme Approach for people with a mental illness referred to specialist mental health services.* Joint Health/Social Services Circular. HC(90)23/LASSL(90)11. London: The Stationery Office.

Department of Health (1990b). The NHS and Community Care Act. London: The Stationery Office.

Department of Health (1993). *Code of practice to the Mental Health Act 1983.* London: The Stationery Office.

Department of Health (1995). *Building Bridges: A guide to arrangements for interagency working for the care and protection of severely mentally ill people.* London: The Stationery Office.

Department of Health (1999a). *National Service Framework for Mental Health: modern standards and service models.* London: The Stationery Office.

Department of Health (1999b). *Effective Care Co-ordination in Mental Health Services – Modernising the Care Programme Approach – A policy booklet.* London: The Stationery Office.

Department of Health (1999c). *Code of practice to the Mental Health Act 1983.* London: The Stationery Office.

Department of Health (2000). *The NHS Plan.* London: The Stationery Office.

Department of Health (2001). *The Journey to Recovery – the Government's Vision for Mental Health Care.* London: The Stationery Office.

Department of Health (2004a). *National Service Framework for Children, Young People and Maternity Services.* London: The Stationery Office.

Department of Health, (2004b). *National Service Framework for Children, Young People and Maternity Services.* London: The Stationery Office.

Department of Health (2008). *Refocusing the Care Programme Approach – Policy and Positive Practice Guidance.* London: The Stationery Office.

Department of Health (2009). *Healthy Children, Safer Communities – Strategy to tackle youth crime/anti-social behaviour.* London: The Stationery Office.

Department of Health (2011). *Early Intervention: the next steps.* The Stationery Office.

Department of Health (2012). *Compassion in practice.* London: The Stationery Office.

Department of Health (2012). *No Health without Mental Health: Implementation Framework.* London: The Stationery Office.

Department of Health (2013). Annual Report of the CMO 2012: Our Children Deserve Better: Prevention Pays www.gov.uk/government/organisations/department-of-health, (Accessed 14 January 2016).

Department of Health, NHS England (2015). *Future in mind: Promoting, protecting and improving our children and young people's mental health and wellbeing.* The Stationery Office.

Department of Justice (2013). *Age of Criminal Responsibility Bill.*

Green , H., McGinnity A., Meltzer, H. et al. (2005). *Mental Health of Children and Young People in Great Britain, 2004. A survey by the Office for National Statistics*. Hampshire: Palgrave Macmillan.

Fowler, J. (1996). The organization of clinical supervision within the nursing profession: A review of the literature. *Journal of Advanced Nursing,* 23 (3), 471–478.

The Francis Inquiry (2013). London: The Stationery Office. HC 497.

Hovish, K (2012). Transition Experiences of Mental Health Service Users, Parents, and Professionals in the United Kingdom: A Qualitative Study. *Psychiatric Rehabilitation Journal (1095-158X),* 35 (3), p. 251.

Hoyle, D (2008). Problematizing Every Child Matters', the encyclopaedia of informal education. www.infed.org/socialwork/every_child_matters_a_critique.html, (Accessed 7 February 2016).

Monitor (2013). Closing the Gap: Better Value Health Care for Patients. IRREP: 22/13 Monitor October 2013.

Moran, (2012). What do parents and carers think about routine outcome measures and their use? A focus group study of CAMHS attenders. *Clinical Child Psychology and Psychiatry (1359-1045),* 17 (1), p. 65.

Munro, E. (2008). Lessons from research on decision-making In: Lindsey and Shlonsky (eds) *Child Welfare Research: Advances for Practice and Policy.* Oxford University Press.

Munro, E. (2011). *The Munro Review of Child Protection Final Report: The Child's Journey.* London: Department for Education.

National CAMHS Review Expert Group (2008). Children and Young People in Mind – National CAMHS Review final report.

NSPCC (2015). Neglect: Learning from Case Reviews Briefing.www.nspcc.org.uk/preventing-abuse/child-protection-system/case-reviews/learning/neglect/, (Accessed 18 February 2016).

NSPCC (2015). Health: Learning from Case Reviews Briefing. www.nspcc.org.uk/preventing-abuse/child-protection-system/case-reviews/learning/health/ www.nspcc.org.uk/services-and-resources/research-and-resources/2014/social-workers-knowledge-confidence-child-sexual-abuse/, (Accessed 17 February 2016).

NSPCC (2015). Realising the Potential: Tackling Neglect in Universal Services. www.nspcc.org.uk/globalassets/documents/research-reports/realising-potential-tackling-neglect-universal-services-report.pdf, (Accessed 2 June 2016).

NSPCC (2014). Social Workers' Knowledge and Confidence when Working with Cases of Child Sexual Abuse.

NSPCC (2014). NSPCC Factsheet: Assessing Children and Families. www.nspcc.org.uk/globalassets/documents/information-service/factsheet-assessing-children-families.pdf, (Accessed 2 June 2016).

Parry-Langdon, N. (ed.) (2008). Three Years On: Survey of the development and emotional well-being of children and young people. Cardiff: ONS.

Proctor B. (1991). Supervision: a cooperative exercise in accountability. In: *Enabling and Ensuring: Supervision in Practice*, pp. 50–57. National Youth Bureau and Council for Education and Training in Youth and Community Work, Leicester.

Read, J. and Reynolds, J. (eds) (1996) Speaking our Minds@ an Anthology London The Open University.

Ronzoni, P (2012). Children, adolescents and their carers' expectations of child and adolescent mental health services (CAMHS). *International Journal of Social Psychiatry* (0020 eds 7640), 58 (3), p. 328.

Schön, D.A. (1983). *The Reflective Practitioner: How Professionals Think in Action*. London: Temple Smith.

Teggart, T. and Linden, M. (2006). Investigating service users' and carers' views of Child and Adolescent Mental Health Service in Northern Ireland. *Child Care in Practice*, 12, 27–41.

Timimi, S (2013). Outcome Orientated Child and Adolescent Mental Health Services (OO-CAMHS): A whole service model. *Clinical Child Psychology and Psychiatry (1359–1045)*, 18 (2), p. 169.

Worrall-Davies, A. (2008). Barriers and facilitators to children's and young people's views affecting CAMHS planning and delivery. *Child and Adolescent Mental Health*, 13 (1), 16–18.

YoungMinds (2013) Same Old... The experiences of young offenders with mental health needs. www.youngminds.org.uk/assets/0000/9472/Barrow_Cadbury_Report.pdf, (Accessed 15 February 2016).

INDEX